One Lump or Two?

A Humourous Story Of One Man's Fight
Against Testicular Cancer

To Hayley

" You must be nuts
to buy this "

Many Thanks

By Darren Couchman

Available from Discovered Authors Online –
All major online retailers and available to order through all UK bookshops

Or contact:

Books
Discovered Authors
Roslin Road, London
W3 8DH

0844 800 5214
books@discoveredauthors.co.uk
www.discoveredauthors.co.uk

Printed in the UK by BookForceUK. (BFUK)
BFUK policy is to use papers that are natural, renewable and recyclable
products and made from wood grown in sustainable forests wherever
possible

BookForce UK Ltd.
Roslin Road, London
W3 8DH

www.bookforce.co.uk

Acknowledgements

Thanks to my Mum and Dad for getting jiggy in the autumn months of 1972, otherwise I wouldn't be here now sharing my experience of testicular cancer.

Many thanks to my lovely wife Sarah and my two gorgeous kids Leah and Charlie. They have stood by me through thick and thin.

Also thanks to my sisters Denise and Lee and my twin brother James. All have helped me through the good and bad times.

A big thank you to Cancer Research UK and DIPEX who helped me achieve my goal of raising awareness of testicular cancer.

Cheers to my mate Dicky Miller who has helped me enormously in getting my book finished. I owe you a pint mate.

A huge thanks to Joe Cole and Lawrence Barraclough for taking the time to write forewords for my book.

Thanks to Stacy Sheppard for setting up my website free of charge. To hire this website wizard for free please visit the website www.youmustbejoking.com

Huge thanks to Jeremy Kenton who has worked tirelessly in helping me raise awareness of testicular cancer through my book. I wouldn't have achieved half as much without this man's help. A true gentleman. Thanks also to his good wife Sharon who makes a blinding sausage casserole.

Many thanks to Daniella Zuccala for helping me with some ideas on my book. Daniella's a student and actually did this for free, yes free. I can't believe it myself. A student doing something for nothing. Miracles do happen.

Lastly thanks to all my family and friends who have supported me over the last seven years.

*This book is dedicated to my
Mum and Dad and to every other person
and their families who have had to deal
with the
terrible effects of cancer*

Foreword
by Joe Cole
(Chelsea and England Footballer)

Testicular cancer is the commonest form of cancer that affects young men, mainly between the ages of 25 and 35.

I am in this age group and I take my health very seriously. That's why I regularly check myself for any lumps and bumps.

Testicular cancer is often seen as an embarrassing illness because of what it affects. There are many men out there who do find something down below, but then are too afraid to go and see their doctor. Unfortunately, if the lump turns out to be something serious, it's often a case of too little too late.

After reading Darren's story you will understand why you need to act fast. I know that if I found a lump down below, I would be straight down my doctors to get it checked out. If you do feel embarrassed, then do what Darren did. Laugh and smile your way through it. By using humour, Darren gets a very important message across to us men. That testicular cancer is not an embarrassing illness at all.

So my advice is simple. Keep an eye on your balls.

Joe Cole

Foreword
by Lawrence Barraclough
(film and documentary maker)

After I made my film 'My Penis and I', the same comment kept coming back to me; 'He might have a small penis, but he's got big balls!'
Well *I* think that although Darren has only got one ball, it's bigger than the pair of mine put together.

The conclusion I have come to after speaking to hundreds of men from all around the world, is that men don't talk about the things that they should talk about: like their feelings or their health. And when they finally do talk about important things, it is often too late.
It's like an unspoken rule.
So men can read about looking after their hair, getting a six-pack and buy a whole range of skin care products to show their feminine side, but that is just the surface.
Can you tell your mate that you're worried that your girlfriend is going to leave you, or that you have a lump on your body you are worried sick about and you think could be cancer? Of course not.

Women talk to each other about anything and everything, so the magazines are full of women's health articles like: 'I think I have a Sexually Transmitted Disease,' or 'How To Check For Breast Cancer.'
It's harder for men to find out about health issues relating

9

to them when Men's magazines are traditionally pre-occupied with cars, gadgets, breasts and football.

So if you're a man worried about a lump or a growth in your lower regions, what do you do? You ignore it and hope it goes away. Why?
Because you're embarrassed and scared to find out, and that's *before* you know for certain you have cancer.

It's an awful thought, but men usually find out they have cancer when it has already reached it's advanced stages. In other words, they are a lot more likely to die from it than women, who are a lot more clued up about medical matters because they talk to their friends and they read other people's medical experiences in women's magazines.

Despite the fact that at times he must have been terrified, Darren has dealt with his experiences with a combination of wit, charm and a laddish sense of humour that reminds you that Darren is an ordinary guy. He could be you.

Darren also asked me to give him a quote to put on the back of his book. I said 'Every man needs to read this book.' Actually, I think that this book should be serialised, with a chapter a day printed in the Mirror.
That way, the message will be well and truly out there and less easy to ignore.

Lawrence Barraclough

Introduction
by Darren Couchman

Is cancer funny? That's a good question. How often do we associate cancer with death and misery? Most of the time. How often do we associate cancer with laughing and smiling? Not often. However, I discovered that laughter is the best form of medicine when dealing with cancer. But when you write a story about living with cancer, it's impossible not to write about the emotional turmoil that goes with it.

So, before you start reading my story, I just want to point out that there's a part of it that isn't funny. It's the part when I talk openly about my Mum and Dad's own fight against cancer and how, in the end, cancer took them away from me. Yes there are parts in the book relating to my own fight that aren't funny, but I will always try to brighten these times up with humour and hopefully you'll see the lighter side of these times.

Yes I know the front cover states, "A Humorous Story Of One Man's Fight Against Testicular Cancer," and that you may well have brought the book because you fancy a laugh and you don't want any emotional crap to go with it. That's good. Thank you. I truly hope you do find my story funny. However, cancer in most people's eyes isn't a bundle of laughs and with cancer comes sadness.

That's fact, not fiction. I can't write a book about cancer and not have any emotion in it can I? It's important that this part of my life is included in the book. Talking about what cancer can do to a family is important. It raises awareness of this awful disease and helps charities gain much needed financial help in their quest to find a cure.

The chapter about my Mum and Dad is at the end of the book, even though this part of my life happened some years before I was diagnosed with testicular cancer. Now I've put it at the end because, to be honest, I don't want to depress you and make you feel down as soon as you pick up the book and start reading it. My story is meant to be funny not sad. I want you to hopefully laugh from the beginning, not depress you straight away and make you say, "He said it was funny, well I'm not laughing." Have a laugh first and then finish with sadness. That's how my sex life works. My wife starts by laughing at my nob and I end up all sad.

However, there is also another reason why there's sadness in the book. It's to help you blokes out there get a shag. So, to all you blokes who have just said, "Shit, I can't believe I brought a book with emotion in it," you'd better take this back immediately. Women love emotion. Now here's what you do. A tip from me. Get your partner, wife, lover or regular swinging buddy to read the book (to be honest this book isn't just for blokes. I'm sure the ladies will enjoy it as well). Hopefully, after reading the final chapter, your good lady will feel really down. They'll need a cuddle. They'll want to feel loved and needed. Bingo. Get in there and give her one. That way she'll feel loved (hopefully not just shagged senseless. Remember lads, when a lady is down its called making love). Then tell her to get you a cold beer from the fridge and this will make her feel needed. There job done. Everyone's happy. The women have had their daily fix of emotion and the bloke has got his leg over. However, please note fellas, I will not be held responsible if you don't get a bit. Don't blame me. I can't help it if your partner hates you or thinks you are shit in the sack. Or that you may have put on weight and become an ugly fucker. You may smuggle a chipolata down your pants on a daily basis. Whatever. It's not my fault. This book isn't a miracle cure to guarantee you a bit of humpty dumpty. You need to explore other options to get your sex life back on track. Like prostitutes for example. So I don't want to see anyone in the small claims court saying, "Darren said that if I got my bird to read this book I'd get a shag. The lying bastard."

Anyway, I hope you understand why I have decided to write my story in this order. Right then, lets get on with it shall we. I hope you laugh your bollocks off. Or your tits. I'm not fussy.

PS. if anything in my book offends you, then I apologise. It's all said in jest and I have no problem at all with the NHS, old age pensioners, the French, women's periods, doctors receptionists, the London Underground, the church..............................

Chapter 1
Man or Woman

It's the year 2000. It's a typical evening in a typical family household. I'm a typical 27-year-old man who's just got in from work, had his tea, played with the kids and watched the twenty-five soaps that occupy the entire television schedule for that night. Now I need to freshen up after a long hard day.

I decide to run a bath and have a relaxing evening surrounded by the wonderful fragrance of our local supermarket's bubble bath. It's supposed to smell of freshly mown grass. It actually smells like the grass has some dog shit in it. Oh well, just get on with it and start relaxing I say to myself. Well I say relaxing. Charlie, my son, has decided he needs a poo at exactly the precise moment I'm about to step into my fragrant bath water containing essence of Labrador shit. Before I can get into the bath I need to wipe his bum. He's only three years old you see. Jesus it stinks, and this goes a long way to ruining the whole ambience of it all. Not even the lit scented candles can mask his awful smell. Yes I light candles whilst having a bath. What's wrong with that? Christ, we're not living in the dark ages now. Actually, that's not a good phrase to use is it? They only had candles in the dark ages and probably lit hundreds whilst having a soak. What I'm trying to say is that we live in the age where men are exploring their feminine side more. I try to explore my wife's feminine side but she won't let me touch it, hence I explore my own instead.

I decide on giving the room a quick spray of air freshener. My finger holds down the spray for at least 10 seconds, trying desperately to cover up Charlie's aroma. I'm now choking on that really awful mixture of stinking shit and air freshener. Mixed together it's a lethal combination. Perhaps this is what the Germans used during the war. A few minutes later I can see the bathroom again, as the thick yellow gas like substance drifts out through the open windows. I'm on my own at last. However, I am not allowed to lock the door in case of emergencies. Like Charlie needing a dump for example!

Whilst I'm on the subject of kids and toilets, I want to have a right old rant about something that really pisses me off. As you read my story you'll notice that I digress every now and again and I'll have a right good moan about things that get on my nerves. We all like to have a moan don't we? Get things off our chest. Well I do.

Right, kids and toilets. Have you seen that bloody advert for toilet air freshener, where the little Chinese kid is having a poo? If you haven't seen it then you can't own a television. Or you must actually have a life and go out every night. Or you are a bookworm and never watch TV. Well, whatever. If you've never seen it please bear with me. Right, where was I? Oh yes, the Chinese boy is having a poo. It must really stink, so he decides to release some air freshener into the atmosphere. However, none comes out, so he promptly says in a really annoying voice,

"It's gone, it's gone."

His mother then sweetly enquires as to what's gone. I've noticed her words aren't in sync with her mouth movements. It's one of them bloody dubbed adverts. How they get away with this I will never know?

He then draws a picture of the empty air freshener on a sheet of A4 paper and slides it under the door for his Mum to see. Now when was the last time your kids went for a crap and took a pencil and a sketchpad in with them? Never, unless they are doing an abstract piece of art entitled, "Toilet paper and poo." It doesn't make sense to me. Mind you, this is the best bit. For him to slide the paper under the door, he must've got off the toilet and waddled over to it. Now, we know he has done a poo because he tried to spray some air freshener to cover up the smell. The question is, "Has he wiped his bum before he takes the few steps to the door?" I reckon not. At the end of the advert the little sod is sitting back on the toilet again, trousers and pants around his ankles, finishing his poo. Which must have meant he waddled a few yards with crap caked around his bum. Dirty little sod. The advert beggars belief. It has got to be the most annoying one I have ever seen. Mind you, the people who thought this advert up must be laughing. The idea of an advert is to make people remember it for years to come. Well it has bloody worked. I want the head of the person in charge of these marketing gits. I want it placed on a spike at Traitors Gate in the Tower of London. This person is a traitor to all normal and decent adverts. Shame on you, who ever you are.

Now, if I were in charge of making this advert, I'd do it like this and make it true to life.

A twenty-five stone man is having a dump. He had a chicken vindaloo the night before. He's sitting on the toilet doing the crossword from "Thai Brides Monthly." The camera pans around the room and we catch a glimpse of the infamous knitted crochet toilet roll cover in the shape of a doll. We then see the toilet brush, now displaying a nice chestnut brown colour around the bristles. He's dropped his load and to be fair it's a stinker. He tries to release the air freshener, but nothing comes out.

He then shouts out to his Thai wife,

"The fricking air freshener has all gone. I'm telling

you, it's all fricking gone."

"Wha has gone me lively hubsand," his Thai wife replies. (No I haven't spelt lovely or husband wrong, I'm just trying to make her words sound like a Thai bird. Okay!).

He then tears off a piece of the magazine and starts to write her a shopping list, which includes a new refill for the air freshener. He gets off the bog and waddles over to the door with his pants around his ankles. Whilst he is doing this, poo is dripping from his bum and making a nice pattern on the grey carpet. He slides the paper under the door and shouts,

"Get down to the supermarket my lovely Internet bride and buy a refill for the air freshener. Oh, and don't forget my case of Stella."

An hour later she arrives back home and makes her way upstairs to the bog. In she goes, replaces the air freshener and gives it a quick spray. Sheer bliss. The advert ends with him still on the bog and drinking a can of Stella, whilst his wife is cleaning the bath and pulling out a mass of hair from the plughole. That's my advert and that's bloody real life. I think I'll start up a campaign to get my one on TV. What do you think?

Right, where was I? Oh yes. I can now do what any normal bloke does in the bath. No, not wash or clean myself, but fiddle with my knackers. As I'm fiddling and rolling my right bollock (the same technique used in the art of play dough), I feel a slight lump. Not a lump attached to my testicle, but a hard stone like lump within it. That's not right I thought. I felt my other bollock, so as not to leave it out, and this one felt normal. I've always checked myself regularly ever since my Mum and Dad died of cancer when I was nineteen. Christ, the luck my

18

family have had with cancer meant I wasn't taking any chances. My bollocks were checked daily and I also led a healthy lifestyle to reduce the chances of any type of cancer growing inside me. Like having salad with my kebab for example.

I now adopted the approach of most blokes in the world and said to myself,

"It's nothing to worry about."

So to stop me worrying about my bollock, I became a woman. Yes, you've heard me right. A woman. I pushed my meat and two veg between my legs and hey presto, a vagina appeared.

Granted it's not the best I've ever seen and blimey it needs a short back and sides before I slip on my red Marks and Spencer thong. STOP!!!!!! I'm getting carried away. However, by doing this remarkable procedure and producing a fanny, I have no bollock and no lump to worry about. There, problem sorted, until my wife Sarah walks in with my daughter Leah to brush their teeth and comments "perv." Sarah said this comment not Leah I must add. Leah was only five at the time and wouldn't know what perv meant. She's too young. Instead she just said,

"So you're a transsexual now then Daddy?"

Kids grow up so quick don't they. My nob instantly springs back into place, albeit a little crumpled and redder than my M & S thong. I tell you what though; this penis and man breast thing just doesn't look or feel right. I reckon I looked far more proportionate when I had my vagina. Anyway, that's enough about my feminine side.

I said to Sarah, "I've got a lump."
"I know," she giggled. " When's it due?"

Yes I have a nice round gut, but I don't care. As I said earlier, if I can't see my bollocks then maybe the lump will go away. My gut is an ideal tool to help me achieve this as it constantly sticks out a mile. I have heard an old wives tale that says your dick doesn't grow in the shade. Judging by the size of my nob, this must have meant I had a fat gut from the day I was born!

" Have a feel Sarah," I ordered.

"Where's the lump?" Sarah said inquisitively.

"On my bollock," I answered.

"Feel your bollock, no way!" she said quite scared.

"Oh yes, I forgot we're married..." I said sarcastically. "What if we role-play and you pretend to be a nurse?" I said applauding my idea, " You can feel it then!"

The bathroom door slammed shut and I just made out the word "off" trailing into the distance.

I got out of the bath, dried myself off, moisturised my face and legs, plucked my eyebrows, poured a glass of wine (a vintage Blue Nun) and started to read July's edition of Take a Break. As I said, I like to get in touch with my feminine side every now and again. Okay I'm lying. It was Cosmo, not Take a Break, but the rest is true!

I went downstairs and explained to Sarah exactly where the lump was, how it felt and that I was confident it would go away in a couple of weeks and I wouldn't need to bother the Doctor.

Yes, that was my game plan. A lump, no, not me. Probably got a knock playing football and the swelling will go down soon. Shame the swelling didn't spread upstairs to Mr Nob.

Anyway, there can't be anything wrong with my privates. It's fathered two kids and always works well in my opinion. I don't need to see the Doctor and that's that.

Now many blokes use this game plan and it actually means in plain English, "I'm not getting my nob out in the Doctor's surgery."

With us men, this fear has been going on since Doctors surgeries were formed.

I think you agree my fellow blokes, that getting your weener out for the Doc to have a look at is a big no no.

Well I know it's my bollock he needs to look at, but the trouble is he cannot just put his hands down my pants and have a rummage around. "Why?" you may ask. Well, firstly it's a bit pervy and secondly I reckon it's illegal. Basically he needs to see my whole package.

"He must have seen a thousand willies all different shapes and sizes," Sarah said quite matter of fact, trying to put my mind at rest.

"Why would he think yours is any different? He isn't going to laugh at it is he?" she added, but with a lack of confidence.

"But you laugh at it. You take the piss out of it. You call it a Walnut Whip," I said, now very emotional.

Most of you must know what a Walnut Whip is. It's that chocolate treat that comes in a blue or red wrapper. It's a shrivelled little treat about 2 inches high with a nut on top. Very delicious though.

Why my missus reckons my nob looks like a Walnut Whip is beyond me. Christ, for a start my nuts are either side of my treat and not on top. Also my nob has never and is unlikely to ever have any chocolate on it for many years to come, even though every Christmas I drop hints and buy Sarah some body chocolate. Every Christmas I lay on the bed naked, waiting for Sarah to baste me in chocolate. Instead she just watches Eastenders and eats the chocolate from the jar with her fingers. Great.

This goes back to the marriage thing I mentioned earlier. Everything stops when you get hitched. You just don't do adventurous things like this when you are married do you? However, I have to say that my nob is tasty, so this is probably why Sarah calls it a Walnut Whip. Nothing to do with the size at all (okay, I'm just saying this to make me feel better).

Tell a lie, there was one time when Mr Nob briefly flirted with some chocolate.

I was sitting watching Men and Motors in my boxer shorts whilst eating a Flake. Bloody hell, they are the crumbliest chocolate bars ever. Loads of chocolate fell through the front opening of my boxer shorts and nestled neatly on my nob. At this point I felt an idea come into my head that could re-ignite the sexual desires in my wife. Sarah loves chocolate and she loves Walnut Whips. What a scorcher of an idea. Pleasure for both of us! Trouble is, it never materialised. Why? Well I love chocolate too and Match Of The Day was on in two minutes. What an evening I had, though I did pull a muscle in my neck trying to get to the chocolate!

Anyway, after a few weeks of deliberating, I finally made an appointment to see the Doctor. The lump hadn't gone away, however I was still scared about getting my package out. What I needed to do was allay any fears I had about how my weener would look when I got it out. So I convinced myself that my nob was an area of outstanding natural beauty and would be looked after forever more by the National Trust. Confidence was high.

My appointment was right after work and to be honest

it would be touch and go as to whether I would make it in time. This was the only time available; otherwise it would be another week of waiting. I asked my boss if I could have a shorter lunch and leave earlier. Luckily she agreed. Now I wouldn't have to rush so much.

Guess what sodding happened? The car wouldn't start. Bugger. I had planned to have a very quick shower at home and then go on to the Doctors. There was no way I was getting my credentials out after eight hours of solid hard graft. No, my nob had to smell of Sphinx (Egyptian Spice) shower gel. It's a cheap imitation of the best selling shower gel for men. I brought it at my local car boot sale. Sarah reckons it makes me smell like a dead mummy! Of course I disagree. I reckon I smell like an Egyptian Prince. Anyway, where was I. Oh yes, the car wouldn't start.

Luckily, I had parked outside a garage and some kind bloke who worked there helped me jump-start my car. Off I went, but now I was running late.

I phoned the Doctors to say I would be running about 15 minutes late and, because of the nature of my appointment, would Doc still see me?

"Of course," the receptionist replied.

I got home with no time for a shower, so I did the next best thing. I whipped down my trousers, pulled down my under crackers and proceeded to lather up my crown jewels with some luxury hand wash.

I know its not Sphinx shower gel, but its nice enough. I mean, has your nob or fanny ever smelt of coconut and mango before? Try it!

I arrived at the Doctors slightly late, but feeling very fresh and tropical in my genital area.

I reported in to reception and waited my turn.

At my Doctors they have an electronic board up on the wall. When it's your turn the board bleeps and your name is beautifully displayed in red L.E.D. lights. It even tells you what room number to go to. Classy.

My nerves were going haywire and I started to get anxious. I was sweating all over. Bloody waste of time lathering up earlier I thought.

I expected the electronic board to bleep and say, "Mr Walnut Whip to room 2." Confidence in my nob was at an all time low, even though the National Trust had placed my nob in the top three most beautiful things in England. Well, when I say England I mean Essex. Actually not quite Essex either. Try Clacton on Sea. Okay I'm lying. Try my house in Little Clacton. And yes the National Trust wouldn't be remotely interested in my area of outstanding natural beauty. I've lied again. So basically my nob is in the top three most beautiful things in my house according to me. What's wrong with that?

"What are the other two most beautiful things in your house?" I hear you cry.

Well, what do you reckon? The two people that bring me joy and happiness and I love with all my heart. No, not my kids. My bollocks! I digress again. Back to the Doctor's surgery we go.

I know he's going to laugh. Then he'll tell the other Doctors and then the receptionists. I'll never be able to come back after today. The receptionists will giggle every time I come in. On the counter there is a box of sweets to raise money for Great Ormond Street Hospital. A box of Walnut Whips will replace these instead. Aaargh!

The board bleeps and strangely it just says, "Mr Darren Couchman, room 2." Not a bad start I thought.

I knocked on the door, entered, and Doc pleasantly greeted me.

24

"What's the problem Mr Couchman?" he asked.

I wanted to say that there was nothing wrong and that I only came in to see if he wanted to join the National Trust, as he'll get a reduced entry price to see my area of outstanding natural beauty. Reduced entry indeed. He's going to see it for free in a minute. Right, no more lies. Just be straight with him I thought.

"I have a lump in my right testicle," I replied.

Strange how all of a sudden I'm polite and using technical terms.

"Right, take down your trousers and pants Mr Couchman and then lay down on the couch for me please," Doc said.

This is it I thought. The moment of truth. He's going to be the new world record holder for the loudest laugh.

I lay down on the couch and he entered through the curtain.

Guess what? He didn't laugh. He was very professional. I could only conclude that either he has seen thousands of nobs before of all shapes and sizes, or he's got a smaller one than me. I preferred the second option.

My advice is don't be scared about going to the Doctors about your privates (women included). I've been there and got the t-shirt.

Seriously, they are professionals and are more concerned about helping you, rather than laughing at your privates. Anyway that's your partner's job.

However, the best bit of advice I can give you is... don't forget to clean it thoroughly before you go.

Doc was now feeling around, twiddling my bollocks between his thumb and first finger (he was a pucker play dough king).

"Nothing to worry about Mr Couchman, it's probably just a cyst," Doc said.

"But you know about my family history Doc. You treated both my parents. You know there's a history of cancer in the family and I'm certain I've got a lump," I said very scared.

"There is nothing to worry about, I can assure you," he said again with confidence.

So that was that. I left the Doctors with full confidence. I mean, he's an expert and should know what he is talking about.

I went back again in a couple of months, as the lump still hadn't gone away and it felt even bigger. Again, the same Doctor said there was nothing to worry about.

Six to eight months after my first appointment I decided to get a second opinion from a different Doctor. I felt something wasn't right and more importantly the lump was still there.

This Doctor didn't laugh either as I pulled down my pants. He must have a small nob too.

He examined me thoroughly. At this time I need to point out that this Doctor has never come across play dough.

"I feel you have a blocked urinal gland," Doc stated.

"Well I'm pissing okay," I replied.

"Are your testicles sore," Doc asked.

"They bloody weren't until you started fiddling with them," I said with tears running down my face. Christ you need some play dough for Christmas Doc so you can get some practice in.

"You are obviously concerned about this lump, judging by the number of appointments you have had. I'm going to refer you to see a specialist," Doc said.

At last. Someone has listened to me. A specialist indeed. And because he is a specialist he will be treated to the smell of Sphinx shower gel and not some crappy hand wash gel containing essence of grape and coriander.

Obviously with hindsight I would have pushed to see a specialist from day one. I know my own body and I could sense something wasn't quite right. Basically the Doctors fobbed me off over the last eight months.

To be honest I don't blame the local Doctors. Lumps on bollocks aren't that common in the UK and also blokes are scared to go to the Doctors and get their package out. They probably only see a few blokes each year with lumps on their bollocks and are not experts in this area.

However everyone, including me, has the right to see a specialist for peace of mind. Don't get fobbed off like I did. Push for that appointment. I'm glad I did.

The letter dropped on the mat. It was my appointment to see the specialist in one month's time. Not bad, fairly quick I thought. I felt okay. I was going to get peace of mind shortly.

One week before my appointment, problems arose.

I was doubled up in agony with severe pains in my bollock and groin area. It was totally unbearable. I could hardly walk.

I knew that possible symptoms of testicular cancer were of course a lump, but the other symptoms were pains in the bollock and groin area. Now I was worried.

My appointment couldn't come quick enough I can tell you.

Chapter 2
Betty Swollocks

How did I feel before my appointment? Bloody worried I can tell you. When I received my appointment letter I was fine. However, as the days crept nearer, I became more frightened. The symptoms I was experiencing scared the crap out of me.

Was it cancer?

I'd seen how cancer had affected my Mum and Dad and how, in the end, it had taken their lives. Blimey, this could happen to me.

However, something else bothered me too. I would have to get my nob out again. Okay, so I got past the small nob Doctors, but this bloke is a specialist. He specialises in nobs and bollocks. He's probably hung like a baboon because specialists have special equipment. They always have the best tool for the job!

He's probably got a really thick book of all the types of nobs and bollocks there are in the world. I bet they have all got Latin names like Beastacus or Pork Swordicus.

I can guarantee my shape has never been discovered before and will be called Walnut Whipus!

This bloke lives and breathes nobs and bollocks. Firstly, I must point out that he is married with kids and my statement is purely from a professional point of view, not pleasure. Secondly, he doesn't actually breathe in nobs, it's a matter of speech.

Remember I said in chapter one to clean your pecker before your appointment? Well listen to this.

My appointment was at 2.00pm in the afternoon and I had to go straight there from work. It was a fairly warm, humid day. On this day of all days the air con at work was actually pumping out hot, damp air, instead of cool dry air. Of course this is reversed in the winter and the cool air appears. Bloody useless air con! It never works properly. It was bloody hot at work and I was sweating buckets. Guess where I was sweating the most? Yes you've guessed it; my bollocks and nob were soaking up the mass of sweat racing down stairs from the rest of my body.

"Oh no!" I hear you all cry. "He can't go to his appointment with sweaty bollocks and an odour resembling a fine mature piece of cheddar!"

Too bloody right I wasn't.

However I was ready. That morning I had popped to the car boot sale and bought Sphinx's new deodorant called Global Warming. I thought I would do my bit to reduce pollution.

It bloody worked all right, because no actual spray came out, which in turn meant no crappy chemicals spurting up in the atmosphere making a bigger hole in the ozone layer. Somehow I can't see this new line catching on.

There was only one thing for it. The hand wash gel in the bog at work. At this time I was working for a bank (the one that uses their staff in their adverts). You know the one I mean don't you? These adverts are like Marmite. You either love them or you hate them.

We had a cleaner come in each day at work, however I'm sure she was recently done under the trades description act.

The sink was bloody filthy, however there was some

good news as well as some bad news.

The good news is that one of the other lads at work must have used the lather up method recently. The bad news was I only knew this because there were loads of black curly pubes all over the sink. I don't think he would stoop so low as to piss in the sink, so it must have been the lather up method that produced the black pubes. He regularly goes on lunch time dates, so I concluded that he lathers up before each one. If it's good enough for him then it's good enough for me. I did rinse the sink first though.

The hand wash gel at work has no label on it, so bugger knows what it smells like and what brand it is. We have strict budgets at work so we now buy in bulk.

We used to have Palmolive, but at the last AGM all the shareholders voted to use the cheap crap instead. I reckon the money that is saved is then used to make sure the directors get Jacobs Creek wine at their Christmas party, instead of the cheap shitty stuff supermarkets churn out.

I made sure all the other lads at work were kept busy, so that they wouldn't interrupt me whilst in a lather, so to speak.

I unplugged all the computers. There was no way anyone would come into the bog now. They would all be extremely busy trying to figure out what was wrong with the damn things.

I ventured into the bog.

Squirt. Out came some liquid into my hands. A nice green colour. I rubbed the liquid between my hands first and then applied it to my sweaty credentials. After ten seconds I became slightly concerned. The aroma of the gel hit me. It reminded me of a smell when I was a kid. My bike chain would come off and I would spend hours trying to get the buggar back on. I would then clean my oily hands with a green looking industrial strength hand cleanser (the stuff that is widely used in the world of car mechanics). Of course. That's it. The hand wash gel at work smells similar to industrial strength hand cleanser! I know that smell anywhere. That smell of oil and grease, mixed with strong hand cleanser, brings back such great memories of me mucking about with my bike as a kid. I can smell it even now as I write. But there's a problem. My nob smells like the hands of a car mechanic who's washed them several times after a hard days shift. Then it hit me. Oh shit. I've seen many adult films (really adult ones) with people using industrial strength hand cleanser for other purposes, all because they have run out of KY jelly!

I can't whip my pants down smelling of this. The specialist will think I have been up to other things. I mean he must watch these films too. Surely this is the most fundamental source for him to study nobs and bollocks close up. Lucky git. Or even worse, he might think I have been extra friendly with Bob the mechanic and that I wanted my spark plug seeing to!

There was only one thing for it.

I ran all the way to my appointment; because I would rather the specialist breathe in good old fashioned sweat, from good old fashioned hard work.

If only I had spoken to the other "latherer" at work. I needn't have put myself through this awful situation. Yes he did have a lunch time date, but this time it was with a right ugly bird. He couldn't get out of it, so he decided to use the hand gel at work, hoping the smell would put the girl off. Apparently for all his other dates he just sprays loads of Right Guard on his nob. I made a note of this for future use.

Anyway, the industrial hand cleanser trick didn't work out quite as he had planned. The ugly bird turned out to be a porn star (he said she had a good body, but only ever did shots from the rear so as not to see her face). She'd used industrial strength hand cleanser many times in her movies and was addicted to it! Poor bloke. That was the longest lunch hour he'd ever had.

I arrived at the clinic out of breath and sweating like a fat bloke in a sauna. I reckon I ran a good half a mile to get there.

I'm not moaning about being sweaty, because as I said earlier I wanted to smell of sweat rather than the awful hand wash gel at work.

When I got to the building I couldn't smell it anymore, so the jog must have done the trick.

I checked in with the receptionist and at this point she said with a grin,

"I'm very sorry but the clinic is running a good hour behind."

Receptionists. Like marmite again, you either love them or hate them. In this instance I would use the latter.

They're bloody miserable when things are running smoothly and bloody ecstatic when things are running crap. Why is this?

I will tell you.

Twenty other blokes and myself are here to see the urologist. As I said earlier he deals with nobs and bollocks and the general plumbing of our crown jewels.

Now we are all worried enough with our potential problems down below, but to have to sit around and wait an extra hour is just plain evil.

All kinds of thoughts enter my mind whilst I sit there pondering.

What if? Why? How? Lots of questions materialise.

Then I start to read all the leaflets and notices on the wall. Most of them say things like, "Do you suffer from headaches," or "Do you get out of breath easily."

Because my mind is a scrambled mess and I'm not thinking straight, by the time I'm called for my appointment I think I've got a brain tumour and heart problems as well!

All this is caused by the extra wait, time on my hands to think, and because I've got half the symptoms described in the leaflets and notices around me.

It wasn't until I got home later that day that I realised the headache was caused by the stress of the extra wait and I was out of breath because I ran to my appointment. Silly Sod.

So going back to why receptionists love it when things go crap. Well, whilst I'm sitting around pondering and suffering all the things I mentioned earlier, I'm getting hotter and hotter. The thermostat has deliberately been turned up to maximum; therefore I am sweating more and more with every minute.

This means that the shower or the lather up sessions us blokes undertook before our appointments were now pointless, as we were all going to smell like unwashed vermin.

The receptionists know this and in a perverse kind of way I reckon they get a bloody good giggle from our misfortune.

However I don't care, because I want to sweat loads and loads to hide the awful smell of the hand wash gel.

So Mrs Receptionist, up yours!

Mind you, I wish the NHS would state in my appointment letters that their clinics always run late (believe me, they all do) and that whilst I'm waiting I'm going to sweat my bollocks off.

This would have saved me from running to my appointment and then thinking I was going to have a heart attack!

I looked around the waiting room and all I could see were old blokes. Christ, I'm the youngest one here!

They've all got their wives with them, which makes me the odd one out as I came alone.

Sarah had to pick Leah and Charlie up from school and playgroup.

Why is it that when I'm in a waiting room full of old duffers, all they seem to do is cough?

Just as I'm about to read an informative notice on the wall about condoms, some old git coughs up loads of phlegm (personally I would spell it f-l-e-m), makes a racket like thunder and then blows his nose on his personalised M & S hankie whilst impersonating a woolly mammoth. Bloody hell it was loud. It shook the whole room, dust and debris falling from the ceiling. I didn't finish reading the article on condoms, as I was too busy pulling out old people from underneath the rubble!

I reckon earthquakes are caused by hundreds of old gits all blowing their noses at the same time.

We could use these men to divert any asteroids on a collision course with the earth. We could line them up and get them all to blow their noses together, just as the asteroid is about to enter the atmosphere

The shockwaves would deflect the asteroid away from earth and we would all live happily ever after. These men who were heroes during the two world wars would be heroes again. This would make a great film. Does anyone know the address of Steven Spielberg?

The next noise I hear whilst waiting is a baby crying. Crikey, every time without fail you hear a baby crying in a waiting room. They don't stop, the parents don't know how to stop them and the cry becomes louder and louder. Everyone tries to make the baby laugh by pulling funny faces or making fart noises. It doesn't work. I know because I've been in the same situation. They only stop crying when you leave the building. It's as if every baby wants to get revenge on their parents because Mummy or Daddy left a poo too long in their nappy. They are programmed to cry in a room full of people, pissing everyone off big time and making the parents look like amateurs. They are then programmed to stop as soon as you reach the outside and no one is about. Kids aren't stupid. They know how to manipulate us.

I look around to see if I can spot the baby in question. Hang on though, I'm in a room full of pensioners. How on earth can there be a baby in the room and where the hell is the crying coming from? Suddenly I'm drawn to a speaker up in the corner. That's where the baby cries are coming from.

I stop a nurse as she's walking through and ask her what's the story with the baby crying sound coming from the speaker?

"We have to have a baby crying sound effect in the room. Otherwise it wouldn't feel right would it Sir? After all, this is a Doctors waiting room," the nurse stated.

Stone me; I've heard it all now. She was right though; it did feel like a proper waiting room.

At least the cries gave a feeling of youthfulness to the room. It's like Gods waiting room in here!

I could've sworn at one stage I saw the man from the Co-Op measuring up some old duffer who had fallen asleep. To top it all I heard his wife say, "He's a tight old bastard. Can we have the coffin done out in MDF?"

I was ear wigging the old couple sitting next to me. What shall I call them? I'll try not being too stereotypical. I know, Darby and Joan.

"You must tell the Doctor about your itchiness and the sharp pain you get when you pass water," Joan said.

Does she mean when he drives past a river or when he's pissing?

" Okay," said Darby sternly.

Joan then turns to me and says, "What are you in for young man?"

The bloody cheek of it I thought. Then I decided to be evil. I was going to have a laugh at their expense. That'll teach Joan for sticking her nose in where it's not wanted.

"Me? I'm back for a check up. I had lots of itchiness and sharp pains when I passed water and they had to cut my nob off," I answered.

You should have seen the old boys face!

"Mr Couchman, we are ready for you now," a nurse shouted down the corridor.

At last. I can escape from "Last of the Summer Wine."

This is it. I'm really nervous now. I'm scared at what they are going to find.

"Hello Mr Couchman, take a seat," the urologist said. He continued, "I've got your referral here from your Doctor. Tell me everything that has been going on."

So I did. I told him about Adam and Eve, the dinosaurs, the big bang theory, the ice age and so on. To be honest, I would have thought a man of his intelligence would have known what's been going on. However, it turns out he wanted to know what had been going on with me. Why didn't he say this then?

So I explained everything in detail, ranging from my lump to the severe pains in my bollock and groin.

"Right lets take a look shall we. Take down your trousers and pants," he said.

As I dropped my trousers I realised my pants were sopping wet. The sweat had taken refuge. Bugger I thought. He'll think I've wet myself, but there's nothing I can do about it now.

Oh well, if he needs a urine sample from me, I'll just wring my pants out over a test tube.

He doesn't even notice my pants and goes straight for my bollocks with his hands.

Now credit where credits due. This bloke has got an A+ grade in play dough manoeuvres.

Within about ten seconds he said, "This isn't normal."

Too bloody true Doc. You are twenty years older than me, you're a play dough emperor and you're fiddling with a young blokes sweaty bollocks. You need to get out more. However, he wasn't talking about his career move.

"I believe you may have a tumour Mr Couchman," Doc said with authority.

"A what?" I answered, not quite hearing him properly the first time.

"A tumour. I want to remove it as soon as possible so I can test whether its malignant or non malignant," he replied.

I could just about take in what he had said. I only heard him say the word tumour. This one word left my thoughts in complete disarray.

The urologist kept talking to me, but I couldn't make out what he was saying.

I could see his lips moving and his arms gesticulating, however not one word was registering with me. It's difficult to describe this feeling, but the best way to sum it up is that my head became heavy, I couldn't focus my eyes properly and the only noise I could hear was my own voice inside my head crying out the word "cancer."

"Mr Couchman, did you take in what I have just said?" the urologist asked.

He had to ask it again. I drifted back into the real world at the point he asked the question for a third time.

"Sorry Doc. I'm a bit shocked at what you reckon the lump is. Can you explain it again?" I said nervously.

He told me to take deep breaths and arranged for a nurse to get me a cup of tea.

Good old tea. Always used in a crisis. It calms people down, lets them focus and thoroughly makes everyone feel so much better.

Perhaps drug users should inject tea instead of heroin? Tea could also become the new cure for all minor ailments.

I can see it now when I go to the Doctors. I've got a really bad chesty cough. It's a chest infection.

"So I'll need some antibiotics then," I say to Doc.

"Oh God no," he replies. "Take three spoonfuls of PG Tips each day and you'll feel right as rain in a couple of days."

"What if it doesn't improve after a few days?" I ask.

"Well come back and see me and I'll get you on the Earl Grey instead. However you will need a prescription for this, as Earl Grey is a far stronger tea."

You never know.....

I digress. I took deep breaths and drunk my tea. I was calm now. PG Tips does work!

He explained it all again, quite matter of fact. I'll give

him his due, he made it so clear for me to understand and he didn't use any jargon whatsoever. However, Doc did say it could well be testicular cancer and to prepare myself for the worst.

The gist of it was this. He was pretty confident I had a tumour. I would then go into hospital in around a week to have the tumour removed and possibly my bollock, depending on the size of the tumour. (This procedure is known as an orchidectomy). Doc did say that it's highly likely that I would have to say goodbye to my testicle. However, there was also a tiny chance of it being unlikely that I would lose my testicle, the chance being as tiny as an ant's todger. But there was a small chance and I preferred to think about this option instead. "Be positive," I thought. I want to hang onto my testicle thanks.

They then send the tumour off to the lab to see if it's cancerous or not. When I say send off, I don't mean it's sent off in an envelope and delivered by Federal Express.

Then there are the results of the biopsy. If it's cancerous then I would need some chemotherapy, and if it's not, then all's well that ends well. He said it would take around 2-3 weeks from the day of the operation before I would get the results of the biopsy.

Great, more waiting. This is going to be hell I thought. Not knowing whether I've got testicular cancer or not and having to wait weeks to find out. Okay, I know 2-3 weeks doesn't seem a long time, but when you are waiting for the kind of news I was waiting for, it really drags. I was going to need to keep myself very busy.

I made my mind up that I would go back to work shortly after my op. At the time I was on a training course in Leeds to become a financial adviser for the bank. I had to stay up in Leeds from Monday to Friday. I reckoned this would be ideal for me to take my mind off the forthcoming results. That was my plan. Right, I've taken in everything Doc has said. I surprised myself at this point of how I'd transformed myself from a nervous wreck to a very calm and relaxed human being.

I know the score and I know what's going to happen over the next few weeks.

Doc wanted a urine sample and a blood sample. I wrung out my pants over a specimen jar for the urine sample and made my nose bleed for the blood sample. Of course I'm joking about the nosebleed (and the urine sample), but at the time I was bloody scared of needles and picking my nose seemed the best way to give blood.

My needle phobia stems back to my old school days when the school nurse gave you a jab every year. Why were all the school nurses back in my day about twenty five stone, as hard as nails and nearing retirement? My school nurse had a voice so deep I thought Barry White was giving out the jabs. She also had lots and lots of facial hair. There was one hair in particular that was growing out of a mole on her chin. It was so long I swear one day I saw a money spider do a bungee jump from it!

Rumours were rife that she joined the nursing game after a stint with the circus as the bearded lady. The circus only got rid of her when they discovered an old woman in Ireland who looked like the long lost twin of Santa Claus. Her days as the bearded lady were over upon this new discovery.

Why couldn't we have nurses who looked like Babs Windsor in Carry On Nurse?

I held the specimen jar in one hand and my nob in the other. I tried desperately to fill it up with pee but I couldn't go.

Sods law isn't it? When you need to pee you can't and when you don't want to pee you go all the time.

Especially when footie is on. I always seem to miss the winning goal because I've got to siphon the python.

I kept trying to think of waterfalls and fast flowing rivers to make myself go. After about fifteen minutes of my travels around the Lake District, I dribbled a few drops into the jar.

As soon as I left the clinic later on and was outside, I was desperate for a slash!

I think it's the thought of placing my bell end in a really small jar that makes my piss tubes close up.

I gave the nurse my urine sample and now it was the dreaded blood test.

I rolled up my sleeve and the nurse (who was actually quite attractive and in her mid-thirties) tied a black strap tightly around the top of my arm.

An attractive nurse, in her uniform, inflicting pain. Nice.

As I was drifting off into my own personal fantasy the nurse said, "Just a little prick."

Bugger me I thought. She can tell this from my urine sample! How clever.

She tapped my vein with her fingers and asked me to clench my fist (strangely my arse also clenched at this point). She chose which vein was best and in went the needle. I looked away. However, I must point out that it didn't really hurt. A small sting, but that was it. All done. How easy I thought. But it wasn't done.

The nurse was having trouble getting the needle into my vein. Several times the needle went in and several times it came out with no joy.

I nearly told her about one particular vein us blokes have where blood is constantly rushing through, but I thought better of it.

At last it was done and my arm was bloody sore. How people have acupuncture is beyond me.

Once this was over, and my heartbeat had returned to normal, I looked at the attractive nurse and realised that I knew her from somewhere. I hadn't twigged before.

I enquired politely and she said yes she knew me also. It turned out she was a regular customer in the bank. Oh great. One of my customers has seen my urine and knows all about my bollock. How many colleagues of mine can boast that?

Next time I'll see her will be after my op. I've probably had my bollock removed and my boss will place me in cashier position number one. That's right, number one because I've only got one bollock.

I'll press the buzzer and it will announce loudly, "Cashier number one bollock."

The nurse will approach my till and coolly say, "Shame about your bollock."

My worst nightmare will happen in front of all my customers. You can bet there will be a bloody long queue as well. Aaargh!

I forget about this awful vision and return back to the real world.

The nurse and I have a casual chat about why the interest rates on her savings are crap and then I leave.

Doc says he'll phone me over the next couple of days to let me know when I need to go into hospital.

As I leave I start to feel emotional. Things were so hectic earlier what with the blood test and the urine sample. Now I was outside and on my own. Christ I wish Sarah was with me now. I start to walk back to work. Then the realisation sets in. If I have got cancer then I'm going to die. I've never felt so lonely. I was being positive about me holding onto my bollock, yet trying to be positive about dying is a trifle harder.

I think about the awful times that Mum and Dad went through. The pain they suffered, the tears they cried. Being told the cancer is terminal and knowing they were going to die. What must have they been thinking?

Well I had a bloody good idea because I was thinking the same.

If I die I'm not going to see my kids get married. I'm not going to see my grandchildren born and I'm not going to be able to hug my wife anymore. This is what Mum and Dad must have thought.

They didn't see me get married and they never saw

my children, their grandchildren. They never saw smile on my wedding day and they never saw my sm when Leah and Charlie were born.

I know they are watching from above and have seen all these joyous occasions, but I want them here with me now. I need their support. But I can't turn to them. They are not here anymore. Life is over for them. Will I suffer the same fate?

All I kept thinking is that cancer ripped my family apart like a tornado and now it might happen again.

Where the hell is my guardian angel?

Tears ran down my face. I had to shield myself from passers by so that they wouldn't see this grown man cry.

I also wanted to know more about this fucking testicular cancer that I may have. I turned round and went back into the clinic. I walked towards the information rack.

It was fully stocked with all kinds of leaflets. There were ones on bowel cancer, prostrate cancer, breast cancer, stomach cancer and just about every other cancer you could think of. Every type of cancer except testicular. Where the hell is it?

After ten minutes of looking I came to the sad conclusion that there wasn't one. Great. I might have this bloody awful disease in my body and I know sod all about it. Nothing.

Yes the urologist went into some depth, but he didn't really explain everything about testicular cancer because I may not have it. Why scare me more? And to be honest, I didn't take it all in anyway. But I wanted to get the facts on it. Be prepared just in case. What is it? How treatable is it? Could it spread? What's the survival rate? All these questions I wanted answering; yet there was no information on it. Boy was I pissed off.

I'm absolutely shitting myself and I've nothing to turn to for answers. Surely this can't be right.

ignited something inside of me. I wiped
and I felt angry. I decided in that moment
to make bloody sure no other man has
the same shit that I've just been through. I
to raise awareness of testicular cancer big time.
True, I may not have it, but I was still adamant I would
do something to help others in the future. This part of my
story is covered later on.

I'd heard of the other types of cancer, but the first time
I had heard of testicular cancer was when Doc mentioned
it. It didn't seem to be common like the other types.

I'd never heard of it in my family. I talked to friends
about it, but again it had never been heard of in their
families.

It seemed like an embarrassing cancer due to the
nature of what it affected.

I was angry and upset. I made my way back to work.
I bumped into my boss as I made my way up the stairs to
the staff room to telephone Sarah.

I struggled to explain what had happened. When I
went to say the word tumour I cried uncontrollably.

Telling family and friends about my tumour was
going to be hard. How will they react? What will they
think? Will they think I'm going to die?

The hardest thing I did that day was telling Sarah my
news. I know how emotional she is and I was worried
how she would take it. How would she cope? This fucking
tumour doesn't just affect me; it affects all my family and
friends.

There I was, struggling to find the right words to say
to Sarah and thinking, " This is so hard."

God knows what it will actually be like if I have got
cancer.

Chapter 3
Me and Dads Army

I eventually told Sarah about my tumour later that day. She seemed okay when I told her and this surprised me a little. However, how she felt in private I'll never know. Yes she probably cried, but in front of me she stayed strong and this helped me immensely.

My operation was going to be in a week's time.

I was still training to be a financial adviser for the bank, therefore the week before my operation I decided to continue with the course and travel up to Leeds as normal.

I reckoned it would be best to keep myself occupied, rather than sit at home with time on my hands pondering.

The course worked like this. I spent one week at home studying and then one week up in Leeds on the course. This was over a 12-week period.

My operation was due to be carried out on the week when I would be at home studying. Therefore my cunning plan was this: In the first week I would go up to Leeds as planned. Then during the second week (a study week), I would go into hospital and have my operation. Then, during my recuperation, I could study in hospital and at home. This meant I would be fully prepared and ready to travel up to Leeds again for week 3 of the course. Bingo. Was I being optimistic with the timescales? Of course I was.

I was on the course with a good mate of mine and I would have to back track to another course at a later date if I missed any of it. This would mean I wouldn't know anyone on the new course. I had briefly met all the other course participants and we had built up a nice rapport. I didn't want to upset the apple cart and meet complete strangers all over again.

Besides, my mate and I had plans for lots of drinking in the evenings after a hard days work on the course. I didn't want to miss out on that. Of course we would be studying as well.

Whilst I was in Leeds, I managed to talk to my mate about what was going to happen the following week.

I told him about my tumour, the operation and that I might lose my right bollock.

Now what happened next played a major part in how I would deal with the possibility of being lop- sided, should that happen.

My mate and I were sitting in the bar of the hotel having a pint. I started talking to him about the operation and what life would be like with only one bollock.

Of course my mate was sympathetic and concerned, but because we've known each other a long time and he knows how my sense of humour works, he started to take the piss.

"Hitler has only got one ball," he started to sing loudly and then proceeded to change the word Hitler to my name.

"You tosser," I said to him, but with a smile. Strangely enough it didn't bother me.

"We might have to call you Uncle Bulgaria," he said grinning.

"Why's that then mate?" I asked.

"Because you'll be a Womble (one ball)," he said laughing very loudly, whilst his whole body shook.

I laughed too. After he had calmed down and wiped away the tears of laughter, he then said,

"What do you call a Russian with three testicles?"

"Go on," I said.

"Who'd you nick a bollock off," he shouted, banging his fist on the table, trying to control his laughter. (Say it quick and it sounds like a Russian name.)

I pissed myself laughing too. Tears of joy were streaming from my eyes. Not one of his jokes upset me; instead he had made me laugh about something that only a week earlier was killing me inside.

This was one hell of a turning point and made me realise that, quite possibly, laughter is the best medicine.

When us blokes talk about our nobs and bollocks I believe we like to have a laugh about them. Yes, many blokes are very shy and rarely talk about their privates with their mates. But chuck in a few beers and all of a sudden we can't stop asking each other lots of questions. How big it is? How much girth has it got? How long do we last in the sack?

If the worst was to happen to my bollock then I was going to laugh about it.

I would shout from the rooftops, "Yes I've only got one bollock, but I'm bloody proud!"

Mind you I couldn't laugh all the time, try as I might. There were many times when I couldn't laugh as fear gripped me. As I said earlier cancer is not a funny business. I had already experienced some negative shit on hearing the word tumour. Little did I know that there would be more dark days ahead. Sometimes I'd think back to that night in Leeds with my mate. I'd use this to try and combat all the negativity. More often or not it worked, but not all of the time. Sometimes you can't smile and laugh when dealing with cancer. Just ask anyone who has lost a loved one to it. There's nothing funny about this. However, I wasn't dead yet. My plan was simple. Try and laugh in the face of cancer and not let the bastard get me down. Yes it would be hard, but fighting cancer isn't the easiest task in the world is it?

The week up in Leeds flew by. The time had come for my operation. I packed my bag and off I went to hospital.

Sarah came with me for moral support.

I'd packed all the normal things you need whilst staying in hospital.

This included anti-bacterial spray, anti-bacterial wipes and some latex gloves. Now I've been in hospitals before, when I visited Mum and Dad for example. I know how the cleaners work. Their bloody mops and brooms don't touch the floor as they dance majestically around the wards, whistling a tune from Mary Poppins.

Now don't get me wrong, it's nice to see someone enjoying his or her job, but not if it means they miss some spots of blood on the floor or a trail of shit leading to the bathroom. I'm not exaggerating; I've seen it with my own eyes.

I wasn't taking any chances, so I went fully prepared.

We arrived at the hospital car park and it took a good twenty minutes to find a space. This infuriates me.

The hospital is a bloody big place and caters for a very large population. How many spaces would you think there are in the car park? About six hundred. Bollocks, or should I say bollock. Try less than half of that number. Why oh why? Work it out please Mr Bigshot of the hospital.

The hospital at any one time could have around 700 patients in the wards. Add to that the hundred or so people visiting the outpatients department every day. Then there is the A&E department, which is always full. Don't forget the maternity ward also. Last, but not least, the hundreds of visitors it receives each day. I think you get the picture.

There are around 250 spaces in the car park. This is useless. The maths do not add up. I know that, every other bugger knows that and deep down so do the big shots.

However they do nothing about it. They are in debt like the rest of the NHS and have strict budgets to adhere to. If this country is not careful, the NHS will fall apart in years to come and we will become like America.

I've experienced good and bad treatment from the NHS. Overall the majority has been good.

Our NHS is the envy of all the other people in countries who have to pay for their own private medical insurance. I just pray the Government doesn't balls it up and reduce our health service to rubble. There are too many chiefs and not enough Indians. Too much red tape and too much paperwork. Mind you, it's the same with every big business that exists in this country. Only time will tell if the Government and its chiefs decide to reduce the NHS to nothing. I hope not.

Sarah and I are now walking towards the hospital. It has a strange look about it. What I mean by strange is the colour of it. The hospital is done out in a very ugly green colour. The colour of snot and puke springs to mind. Now I like green, but not on the outside walls of a hospital for God's sake. I'm nervous about the whole op thing and I would like the hospital to be welcoming, not reminding me of greenies and sick. It should be a nice neutral colour. Magnolia I think. Everyone loves Magnolia.

The best bit about walking towards the hospital is the lovely duck pond and picnic area sitting neatly amongst the hospital grounds. It's just before the main entrance. A bridge takes you over the pond and right up to the front door.

Plenty of ducks, geese and moorhens live on the pond. There's nothing more relaxing than feeding the ducks. The NHS got this idea spot on when developing the hospital and its grounds.

My kids love feeding the ducks and to see their faces light up when doing so is sheer bliss. What's even more magical is seeing all the sick kids from the hospital feeding the ducks. I bet they have been through some tough times and been stuck in their beds for weeks. Yet something so simple can light up many a sad face. I can sit and watch these kids for hours and all my worries are lifted in an instant. All because of that joyful combination of children, ducks and bread. It's a bloody cheap day out as well. Mind you, it's weird also. Take my kids for example. Leah and Charlie are feeding the ducks and are pointing out how lovely they all look, especially the baby ducks. Yet the same evening they are tucking into crispy aromatic duck from the Chinese. It's the same when we visit farms. Oh what lovely cows and their calves.

"What do you want for lunch kids?" I ask.

"Beef burger and chips please Dad," they answer.

The cow turns its back on us in disgust and promptly drops half a tonne of shit.

What a funny world we live in.

Anyway back to the story. Sarah and I walk over the bridge towards the main entrance and I swear I heard a duck quack "Good luck."

We are now at the main door to the hospital and then

something hits me. This could be the last time I'm out in the open with two bollocks. What a thought. I then tried to think back to my last shag with two bollocks. That's a momentous part of my life. That will go down in history.

When was it though? Buggar, I can't remember!

"Sarah," I said. "When was our last shag?"

"Shag?" she said in disbelief. "Don't you mean when did we last make love?"

Women eh. Make love. That's when we first started going out, not now we are married! (Unless of course you are married and you're going to roger your wife after she's read the final chapter and is feeling down. Then it's making love. Please remember this important rule from my introduction).

Then I remembered. Of course, it was last year on my birthday!

I walked up to reception, showed the bloke sitting there my appointment letter and I was directed to a room opposite.

"Wait in there mate and a nurse from your ward will come and get you shortly," he said.

Sarah and I sat down in the waiting room. She was glad to take the weight off her feet as she had carried my overnight bag from the car park to reception. Bloody hell, I wasn't going to carry it. I'm the patient here!

There were a few other people in the waiting room, men and women, and they all sat nervously rubbing their hands or looking at their watches every twenty seconds or so.

I didn't say a word to Sarah the whole time we were

in there. No one else said a word either. You could've heard a pin drop or a flea fart.

All of us were caught up in our own little worlds. Everyone had their own reason to worry, husbands and wives included.

I looked at the other nervous people and began to wonder what was going through their minds. Probably the same thoughts as me. We are all in hospital and we all have some kind of illness that needs treating. However, I expect their biggest worry, like mine, was "Am I going to get better?" or "Do I make my peace with God now?"

There was very little eye contact apart from the occasional look up from a bloke opposite me. This look was followed by a nervous smile and a nod. He looked crushed, he looked pale and he looked like the whole world was on his shoulders. Then again he probably thought the same about me, because that's how I felt also.

I know I said I was going to use laughter to get me through the difficult times, however on this occasion and in this atmosphere it didn't feel right. Sometimes in certain situations you just can't drag yourself from the pits of negativity. This was one of them. This was a waiting room full of scared people. I sensed there was a rule saying silence must be observed. Anyone who made a noise would be looked upon with disgust and then promptly killed. We have all drifted away into our little worlds and shame upon the man or women who interrupts our thoughts.

Suddenly the deafly silence was broken by the old man as he blew his nose several times into his hankie. He sounded like an elephant with a trombone stuck up its trunk. He then proceeded to cough a number of times, resulting in a mass of phlegm rising from his throat into his mouth (still reckon it should be spelt f-l-e-m). Everyone looked up suddenly and their eyes fixed upon him instantly. If their eyes were daggers he'd be dead. I felt sorry for him. Not only had he interrupted everyone's

52

thoughts, but he also had a mass of phlegm in his mouth to get rid of. I knew it and so did everyone else. He had the choice of spitting the gob into his hankie for all to see, followed by tuts of disgust, or he could swallow it and bring it to the surface later on in the privacy of his own room.

He took the second option. Nice. Mind you, all credit to him, his face didn't grimace. He swallowed, he smiled, down went his head and then he started rubbing his hands again very nervously.

He's a pro I thought. I must admit I did go a bit goose pimply watching an expert excel in his chosen passion.

Everyone else at this point nodded their heads in approval with his chosen method and carried on with their nervous habits. I was going to give him a standing ovation and shout, "Encore," but I thought better of it. More importantly he had won the crowd back and ensured he would not be dying today after all.

The door opened and in walked a nurse. We all sat up in expectation, hoping she had come for us. We all wanted to escape this horrible atmosphere and boredom and just get on with it. As I've said before, the longer the wait the more nervous I get.

"Mr Couchman, we are ready for you now," the nurse said as she gave me a huge smile.

Nice I thought. Size 12, boobs a 32C. She fitted snugly into her uniform. Please God let this be the nurse who does the bed baths.

As I left the room I looked around. I was pleased I was going to my ward, but at the same time I felt a sense of sadness.

When the nurse had opened the door to come in, you could see everyone getting excited (and not just because her nipples were showing through her uniform). The colour had come back into their pale faces and the weight of the world had been lifted in an instant from upon their shoulders. They sat up expectantly, waiting for the nurse to call them. When they realised it wasn't their time they slouched back into their chairs, their faces became pale again and the world once more perched itself on their shoulders.

Some of these poor buggers would have to go through this ritual many more times before they were called to their wards. Life can be so bloody cruel at times. However, their time was about to get worse.

As I was leaving the room a speaker suddenly came alive and wailed out the most annoying baby cry ever. Poor gits I thought. However this is a waiting room, what do you expect?

"Goodbye comrades," I thought as the door shut. "Think of England."

I followed the nurse down the long winding corridors and up a few flights of stairs. Eventually we arrived at the ward entrance.

"Please would you ensure you wash your hands every time you enter and leave," the nurse said.

There was a dispenser unit on the wall and with a couple of pumps it produces some hand wash gel used to kill all types of bacteria on your hands. This wasn't just ordinary hand wash gel though. No, it was alcohol-based gel. It needs to be strong stuff to combat all the nasty bugs in the world. This stuff was so good it even dried itself, making paper hand towels redundant. Bloody good for the environment. What a cracking invention.

One thing did cross my mind though. This gel contained alcohol. I had visions of all the local piss heads queuing up at weekends, ready to drink from the dispenser. Would it taste like Fosters, or would it taste like dishwater? They all need their weekend alcohol and this free bar in the NHS would be ideal to cater for their needs. Mind you, I have to admit I did try a bit for myself. Purely for research of course to see what lager it tasted like. I can see why I never saw anyone else drinking from it. It tasted like a weak shandy!

We all washed our hands in shandy and the nurse then punched in the security code to open the door. They flung open and in we went.

The ward was very busy. The phone was ringing constantly; nurses were rushing about here and there. The whole atmosphere cried out, "So much to do and so little time to do it."

It was this first impression that made me realise why nurses can get stressed out doing their jobs, whilst earning a wage that in no way is reward for the good work they do.

The nurse showed me to my bed. Bugger. It wasn't a private room, but a bed on the ward. There were eight beds to a bay, four along one wall and the other four exactly opposite.

Men occupied all the beds. This was a men only ward. Now of course you do get mixed wards. However, due to the nature of why us men were in hospital, it's only right that this ward was for blokes only.

I'm sure ladies didn't want to hear me say to the bloke in the next bed,

"How's your cock doing mate?"

Of course ladies have women only wards for the same reason.

"What? Ladies have cocks?" I hear you cry.

No. What I mean is they have women only wards for

women only problems.

Mind you, in some parts of Thailand women do have cocks. I read this in a book and have not experienced this first hand, unlike many unsuspecting fellas in this world who have come across the famous lady-boys, so to speak.

All the blokes, except the one next to me, were old looking. The fella next to me looked around 38 years of age.

We all had one thing in common. We all had something wrong with our packages in some form or another. This was a ward for the waterworks department. Of course all the other men knew this too. I gave them each a friendly nod and they seemed genuinely surprised that a bloke of my age should even be in here.

"Make yourself at home," said the nurse. "The Doctor will be along shortly to see you."

Make myself at home. Damn, I forgot to bring in my Playstation and February's edition of Knockers Monthly.

Sarah, exhausted, put my overnight bag down on the bed. Actually she threw it down.

"Careful," I shouted, "My best bottle of aftershave is in there."

Now as you know lads, Hai Karate isn't cheap.

"You've probably broke my soap on a rope as well," I added.

Yes Hai Karate again. This was a vintage soap on a rope by Hai Karate. An '88 I think.

I thought now was a good time to use this antique Christmas pressie. Show the nurses a bit of class, as they're probably fed up breathing in Brut all the time from the old gits.

As the nurse walked off she shouted back, "Don't forget to put your gown on. It's on your bed."

"But I've got my own pyjamas," I replied. "They're Doctor Who ones."

"No, it's the gown I'm afraid Mr Couchman. It's easier for the Doctor to inspect your testicles," she said.

Jesus, tell everyone why don't you!

"Doctor will be here shortly to have an inspection," she added. "You will also need to keep the gown on when you go down for your op and also when recuperating. The gown provides much easier access than your pyjamas."

"Suppose I'd better get used to it then," I said.

Sarah pulled round the curtains and I began to undress.

The NHS gown is a sight to behold. Bloody awful things.

My gown was an off white colour with blue squares.

You put your arms through the front and it ties up at the back.

Sarah wanted to help me put it on, but I insisted on doing this myself, as there may be many times over the next couple of days where I'll be on my own. I might as well start practising now.

I felt a great sense of achievement as I turned round to Sarah and announced, "All done."

It had taken me around ten minutes. I'd felt like Houdini in a straight jacket, but in reverse as my arms flailed around my back trying to do up the ties and not undo them like Houdini. However, I'd done it. I imagined the applause from all the nurses and other patients. Perhaps I had achieved the quickest time in NHS history, or perhaps the applause was for the fact everyone knew what a sense of achievement it was putting the bloody gown on.

"Well, what do I look like," I said to Sarah.

"Wee Willie Winkie," she replied laughing.

Crikey, there must be a piss flap at the front of the gown and my nob is trying to poke his head out and introduce itself to the entire ward.

Sarah actually meant I looked like Wee Willie Winkie and was not observing my tackle rear its ugly head through the flap.

"You only need a night cap and a candle in your hand," she said, "And then you can run through the town like Wee Willie Winkie."

Yeah, chasing the nurses I thought mischievously. As I was thinking of chasing beautiful nurses through the corridors, my weener suddenly poked its head out from beyond the flap in a state of arousal. It could've stayed inside whilst hard, but oh no, the sod wanted to have a look around. How embarrassing.

Talking of running, I needed a pee and was desperate to go. Sarah pulled back the curtains (she's finished carrying my bag, so she might as well make herself useful) and I proceeded to run towards the bog.
I didn't care what I looked like in my gown, my pee was my priority.
I did a pee and then walked back towards my bed

trying to look like Brad Pitt in a gown.

As I was walking back I noticed some of the nurses laughing and pointing at me.

Then some of the old boys did the same.

I got back to my bed and Sarah was pissing herself laughing too.

"What?" I said puzzled.

"You silly sod. Your bum was showing all the time you were walking," Sarah replied. "You hadn't done the bottom ties up!"

Bugger me I thought. Now, my bum is quite a nice shape, so I haven't got a problem with people staring at it. However, it is hairy and spotty. The spots actually convert to a dot to dot on my bum cheeks. The spots make the letter W on each cheek and when I bend over it spells out the word WoW!

Matron came marching down the ward towards me and boy did she look angry.

"Mr Couchman. When you were asked to strip off and put your gown on, we didn't mean for you to go commando," she said sternly.

Now she tells me.

By now it was lunchtime and the catering lady had arrived with her trolley at my bed.

"I've got macaroni cheese or shepherds pie with some veg," she announced.

What a choice. I hate macaroni cheese, so I opted for the shepherds pie with, I hoped, a melody of winter vegetables.

What I got was a splodge of mince with mash potato on top and some peas. Twenty peas in fact because I counted them.

The portion was hardly enough to fill the stomach of a baby flea, so it would hardly notice in my enormous cavern.

"For afters you can have a yoghurt or peaches with custard," she said in a weary sort of way.

I felt sorry for her because she has to say the same old shit every time she serves a patient. No wonder there isn't any enthusiasm in her voice. She sounds like the women bingo callers you hear in the arcades, their voices droning on and on.

"What flavour yoghurts have you got please?" I asked.

"I haven't," she snapped, "I've run out."

This is what I mean. She's so robotic and repetitive in what she does and says, that she'll say she's got yoghurt when she bloody well knows she hasn't.

"Peaches and custard then please," I said nervously, thinking she might shout back, "Out of that too."
However she had some. She plonked my peaches and custard down on my table next to my tiny portion of shepherd's pie.

"Tea or coffee?" she droned on.

"What one have you got?" I asked, thinking I'll save myself some time and also avoid a sharp bark from her.

"Well I've got both ain't I, otherwise I wouldn't have said so," she snapped back. Bloody typical.

"Coffee please," I answered as I hid behind my

pillow.

She poured it out, slammed it down on my table and spilt half the contents. On she walked, pushing her livelihood along to the next unsuspecting poor bugger.

I looked at my feast. I could hear my stomach crying out, "If you think that's enough fatty, then think again."

I then heard it chant, "Hob Nobs, Hob Nobs."

I sent Sarah down to the hospital shop with a fiver. I wrote down what I wanted on a bit of paper, as her memory is a bit vague. Her mission, which she accepted, was to buy four different varieties of biscuits that would satisfy my hunger. She also had to come back with £2 change. The exact change. I like to set Sarah these tasks now and again. It keeps her brain active.

As Sarah left muttering, "This is a mission impossible you wanker," there was a small explosion as the message I had written self destructed in less than ten seconds. Strange.

I then started on the shepherd's pie. I don't mean I picked on it and wanted a fight, I mean I started to eat it.

Sarah had just finished saying various expletives and my shepherd's pie was gone. Two forkfuls and I had eaten it. Surprisingly it wasn't bad. I've tasted worse (I could write a chapter on Sarah's cooking but I won't).

The peaches and custard were next. Again, not too bad.

I would like to add at this point that the hospital food that I ate over the next few days was fine. I'd heard all sorts of stories about the food before I went in for my op. All negative. I even took with me the takeaway menus for my local kebab house. Credit where credit's due, the catering company were serving up edible nosh. The only down side was the size of the portions.

Again, it's all about keeping the costs down in the NHS. I did have my own theory though. Listen to this:

Sarah came back from the shop. Her shoulders were

slumped and she announced she had failed her mission miserably. Unlike Tom Cruise who always completed his missions. She had only brought 3 packets of biscuits (Hob-Nobs, digestives, and chocolate digestives) and had come back with 50p change. She had failed both parts of her mission.

"£1.50 each the biscuits are!" she said.

"You should've walked to Asda and then you wouldn't have failed your mission," I joked.

She didn't see the funny side and she plonked herself down in the visitor's chair and proceeded to read her copy of Womans Own.

This is my theory. You get small portions of nosh. You're starving. You then spend your hard earned money on extortionately priced biscuits in the shop. Thus the catering firm also owns the shop and rakes in even more profit. There, I've said it.

Is it true? Who knows, but hey, we all like a good conspiracy theory in this country don't we?

The nurse then came to see me and said the Doctor will be about an hour, as he wants to make sure my lunch goes down properly and that I don't get indigestion.

"Is he having a bloody laugh?" I thought. I could hardly get indigestion on portions made for people from Lilliput (a fictional town in Gullivers Travels where little people lived).

As for an hour for my lunch to go down, try thirty seconds Doc!

It was more like two hours before the Doctor came to see me and in between Sarah and I tried to do the crossword in her Womans Own magazine to kill some time. We got stuck into it and after an hour or so we were nearly done.

We had one question left, but we were stuck for the

answer.

The question was,

"Name the actress who always appeared alongside Russ Abbott in the Russ Abbott Show?"

I could see her in my mind, but her name escaped me. Sarah didn't have a clue either. I loved the Russ Abbott show as a kid and I watched it every week, yet I couldn't think of the leading lady's name. Come on man think. She played Blunderwoman. No, it's no use. My brain had gone dead.

At this point a nurse I hadn't seen before entered the ward. A rather large lady with great big knockers. She smiled as she walked by and whistled the theme tune to Dogtanian and the Three Muskerhounds (another favourite programme of mine when I was a kid). For the benefit of any older readers she whistled the theme tune to Z Cars. For any teenage readers she whistled the theme tune to Hollyoaks.

As she passed the other men she would make a joke with them and bellow out an enormous laugh. She looked a right bloody laugh!

"Hey Sarah," I said. "She looks like that bloody Bella Emberg from the Russ Abbot Show."

And that was the rather bizarre moment that enabled us to complete the crossword. Of course, Bella Emberg! I can see her now.

Thank you large nurse. You saved me having sleepless nights, tossing and turning, trying to think of the answer. I owe you a debt of gratitude.

Yes you may carry out a bed bath on me you lucky cow….

Around two hours later the Doctor arrived at my

bedside. Four other people, all carrying clipboards and scribbling down every word the Doctor said, surrounded him.

They all looked about 16 years of age. They were student Doctors. Fresh faced, intelligent looking and very eager to learn. Did they realise though, that once they had qualified (yes they would earn good money and quite rightly so) they would be working extremely long hours. Their social life would be non-existent. I believe you've got to have a healthy work-life balance. I don't think Doctors are able to get this balance right. Yes they do a fantastic job, but hell, they are entitled to a life as well. It's not their fault. It's the demands of the public and the Government that means they only get four or five hours kip a night.

The Doctor was now scanning his notes and he turned to the student Doctors and said, "Right everyone, this is Mr Couchman."

They all looked at me and smiled.

"All right?" I said.

"Mr Couchman has a tumour on his right testicle and tomorrow he will be having his operation to remove it," Doc stated. "We don't know yet if the testicle will also be removed, this is of course dependent on the size of the tumour. However, it's highly likely the testicle will have to be removed also."

Thanks Doc. There's me trying to be positive about saving my testicle and you've said the same as my urologist. That's two of you who think I'm going to live the rest of my life with just one. Anyway, I don't care. I'm still confident I'll wake up from my op with two.

The student Doctors scribbled furiously. Bloody hell I thought. They're making notes about my bollock. They could use me as an example during their lectures, or even write their final dissertation about me entitled, " Mr Couchman's Bollock."

The Doctor by now had whipped around the curtains and asked me to present my tackle for inspection. The student Doctors all gathered round.

Great I thought. Two of the student Doctors were young women, aged about eighteen, and now I've got to show them my nob. What notes will they scribble down?

Probably something like, "Once Mr Couchman has had his op we recommend he comes back for a penis extension," or "The stress of the operation has caused Mr Couchman's penis to shrink into a shrivelled prune and hide between his two testicles."

Now normally if two 18-year-old girls wanted to have a look at my purple-headed warrior it wouldn't be a problem, because I would have an erection and my nob would grow and reach the size that is average across the UK. Which by the way is four inches (yes, four inches). The six inch thing is a myth. No girl is allowed to laugh at this size; otherwise she will be laughing at the majority of British men, including me.

However the problem was this. It would be totally wrong for me to get an erection whilst two female student Doctors looked on. Trouble is, without the erection the girls would probably have trouble seeing it. What shall I do? Jesus Christ you wimp. Just get it out and get on with it. Christ, I'd shown my tackle to several complete strangers over the last eight months or so. How hard could this be? Bloody hard if I decided to think about the female students poking my prick with their fingers. Within seconds my nob would be standing to attention in all its glory. Yes I could do with some blood rushing to my nob and making it look presentable, but at the same time I didn't fancy getting arrested for indecent exposure (even though it would be the girls fault).

Right there was only one thing for it. I'd rather they see my nob in its hibernating state, rather than see my glorious morning marrow!

As I pulled open my gown and whipped down my pants, I needed to think of something that ensured no blood would rush to my throbbing vein.

What could I think of to ensure a lifeless shrivel of foreskin? Then it came to me. I'd think of me shagging an old granny with saggy tits, whilst her husband spanked my arse with his solid oak walking stick. This image is bound to keep the old pecker down.

As Doc felt my bollocks and the female students leant over closer, I thought of this peculiar image.

Oddly enough and rather shamelessly, I have to admit that my pecker started to fill up with blood as I pictured the old granny removing her dentures to perform some French oral!

Quick, I need to think of something else before it gets too hard. I know. Two female Russian weight lifters having a lesbian fight in some rice pudding. It worked a treat. I hate rice pudding and putting two large hairy lesbians from Moscow in it made me feel really sick. The blood stopped in an instant and the relief was unimaginable.

I let out a loud sigh just as Doc was fiddling with my right bollock. Now that was the wrong time to let out a sigh. He looked at me with disgust. He finished his examination as quickly as he had started. He moved swiftly on to the next patient, shaking his head and muttering something about how his hands always tend to arouse the men patients. Don't knock it Doc, it's a gift from God!

Whilst all of this was going on the students were again scribbling down lots of notes and I swear one of them was drawing a bloody picture of my nob. It was either this or the student was bored and was doodling.

I must just say that not one of the students laughed. They acted in a mature and professional manner and asked the Doctor lots of questions as he carried out his examination. Nothing to have worried about after all. They probably didn't even look at my nob and focused more on my bollock instead.

As the students followed the Doctor to the next bed, I heard one of the female students say,

"I don't know why, but I don't half fancy a Walnut Whip."

Bloody Marvellous!

The nurse then came back to see me and said the surgeon would be along shortly to discuss my operation.

Sarah had to go now as Leah and Charlie would need picking up from school and playgroup very soon. This everyday chore now seemed so exciting after being stuck in the visitor's chair for hours on end. She was bored rigid and there's only so many times you can read Womans Own headline story, "I slept with my boyfriend's sister and now I'm a lesbian."

I made sure I had plenty to read whilst I was on my own, although I could listen to the radio via some headphones, which the hospital provided. The trouble was I could only tune in Hospital FM, listening to some boring DJ wannabe playing endless Donny Osmond records. I only listened to it when I needed a kip. It beats popping endless sleeping pills!

There was a television in our bay, but this was shared between me and all the other blokes. I didn't get a look in most of the time. All the old duffers outnumbered me.

Whilst I wanted to watch Richard and Judy, all the old duffers insisted on watching Last Of The Summer

Wine. Mind you, who can blame them? There are lots of old women in this programme for the old gits to fantasise over. I watch the ten-minute free view on satellite to satisfy my sexual urges, yet the old boys prefer Last Of The Summer Wine or Miss Marple!

One old boy opposite found it hard to control himself. A shot appeared of an old woman putting her smalls on the washing line and that was it. He created an instant tent with his sheet due to his sudden arousal. His tent stayed upright through the entire show.

Mind you, as the credits rolled his tent instantly fell back down to earth.

Instead of viagra for the old boys, Doctors should instead prescribe a photograph of an old woman washing and scrubbing her bra and knickers the old fashioned way. It worked for the old boy in my ward and he was about 90 years old!

Right, now that load of old crap has finished it's my turn to watch something half decent. I flicked through the channels and found the Simpsons. I settled back down on my bed and relaxed. What more could a bloke want. Nurses looking after me all day long, the Simpsons are on and I'm nibbling on a Hob Nob. Sheer bliss.

The 38-year-old bloke in the bed next to me nodded approvingly.

"At last, something decent to watch," he said relaxing.

I passed him a Hob Nob so that he too could experience the meaning of the words, "Sheer bliss."

As the Simpsons started, all the old gits united and said,

"What's this useless programme then?"

"It's the Simpsons and it's funny," I replied, "Give it a go."

"Nah," they all said in unison, "We don't want to watch a kids cartoon."

What the hell do they know? Like a synchronised swimming team, they all picked up a magazine, huffed and puffed a bit and then began to read.

Guess what they were reading? "60 plus." Honestly, I'm not lying! It's probably got a centre-spread piece of a naked old woman covering her modesty with a Saga holiday brochure.

Just as the Simpsons got going the bloody surgeon arrived to see me.

He pulled round the curtains, but just before they shut tight I said to the bloke next to me,

"Make sure Dad's Army doesn't turn it over."

"They can bloody try," he replied with both thumbs up, grinning like a Cheshire cat.

"Right then," the surgeon said, "Lets have a chat about your operation tomorrow."

As he finished his sentence two more people walked in through the curtains. They were part of the surgical team.

The surgeon asked me to whip open my gown and pull down my pants. Christ not again. Groundhog day or what?

"Whilst my nob's out, do you want to enquire if all of kingdom come want to have a butchers at it as well? This will save me getting it out again later," I thought.

In the past eight months, complete strangers have seen my nob more times than my own wife. And they had a fiddle with it, which is more than I can say of Sarah!

I opened my gown and down went my pants. Again.

The surgeon explained to me that he would be marking my body with a felt tip pen, this indicating the whereabouts of the incision.

It was when he started to draw a black line just below my right groin that I thought, "What the fuck is he doing?"

I'm in to have a tumour and possibly my bollock removed and this guy is doodling near my groin. This was a good few inches away from my scrotum, so what's he playing at.

"I think you've got the wrong bloke Doc," I said really worried.

He looked at his notes and added,

"No, I don't think so. You are Mr Couchman and you are in to have a tumour removed from your right testicle. Everything's in order," the surgeon replied.

"Then why are you drawing black lines near my groin?" I asked. "Surely to God you just cut open my sack to get to my bollock?"

Christ, I'm not Doctor Dolittle, but even I know this would be the quickest way in.

"No no Mr Couchman, I can't do that," he said. "I have to cut just below your groin and venture downwards to remove the tumour. If I have to remove your testicle, which is highly likely, then I will need to remove some tubes connected to your plumbing. I can only do this by going in from your groin area. Also I need to check and see if the tumour has spread anywhere else. It's all done for your benefit."

"I can see that now," I replied.

Blimey. He's the third person to say it's highly likely I'll lose my bollock. It doesn't matter though. I'm staying positive.

Bloody hell. I thought I'd have a small cut on my sack and be up and about in a couple of days. Probably just be a little sore.

The surgeon then proceeded further. "This isn't a minor operation Mr Couchman. It's fairly major and you should allow yourself around 2-3 weeks to recover."

Bugger that. I wanted to be back at work in Leeds the following week. I was adamant I would be okay. I'm a quick healer!

The op would be around one o'clock tomorrow afternoon. This meant I had to fast from that evening. I would miss Tuesdays breakfast and lunch. Even nibbling on my Hob Nobs was a no no.

The surgeon explained that a porter would come and get me and take me down to theatre. Great! A bit of entertainment before I go under the knife! What was on? Phantom of the Opera or The Lion King? I hope it is Joseph and His Amazing Technicolor Dreamcoat.

"If I do have to remove your testicle Mr Couchman, which is highly likely, then please be assured that in no way does anything change. You can still lead a normal healthy life with just one testicle," the surgeon said with confidence.

The surgeon has said "highly likely" again. If I hear those words again, then it's highly likely I'll shit myself.

"Fair enough," I replied. However, I didn't have confidence in his words. A normal healthy life my arse.

Surely if I've only got one bollock this is going to affect my sex life, albeit I'd only have to worry about this once a year! From the day the specialist told me that they might have to remove my testicle, I didn't really think about spending the rest of my life with one bollock. As I said before, I'd assured myself that this couldn't possibly happen. There was still that teeny weeny chance I'd keep it. Trouble is the surgeon had said the same thing as the urologist and the Doctor. Now I wasn't so sure. Fingers crossed they don't. Better still, legs crossed they don't!

The anaesthetist would then be the next person to greet me. He or she would then give me the anaesthetic and I would be away with the fairies.

The op would last around three quarters of an hour to an hour.

I would then be taken to the recovery unit to recover. Obviously. What else could I do in a recovery unit apart from recover?

Once I'd come back round I would then be assessed to make sure everything was okay. Once I got the all clear I would then be taken back to my ward and hopefully go home the next day.

Excellent. The surgeon had explained every detail blow by blow. I knew exactly what would be happening at each stage of my journey.

"Thanks Doctor," I said as he walked off, "See you tomorrow."

I had my final supper that evening (well you never know with operations). Mind you, if this was to be my final supper then what a shit one it was. I wanted chicken in a white wine sauce with sautéed potatoes and mange tout. I got sausage and chips. Great.

As I was fasting that evening I did ask for extra portions. It was a different lady to earlier and I think she had the hots for me as she gave me an extra sausage. And it was a jumbo one!

It still didn't fill me up though, so I munched my way through two packets of biscuits before the dreaded time of six o'clock arrived. This was the time I had to start fasting.

I ate the biscuits so quick that I ended up with loads of crumbs in my bed. There's nothing worse than laying on your bed amongst lots and lots of crumbs. My arse and nob instantly became crumb magnets.

Bloody hell, I'll have to have a shower in the morning now. There's no way I'm going to let the surgeon see my nob covered in crumbs impersonating a digestive. Christ, he might bloody eat it!

Chapter 4
Five, four, three, two, one...

I woke up the next morning looking forward to my breakfast. Then I realised I wasn't allowed one. Bugger. I was starving!

This fasting lark is bloody hard, especially when I am used to big meals.

How the Muslims fast during their religious festival Ramadan is beyond me. I have the utmost total respect for their religious beliefs. I couldn't do it.

Mind you, there are plenty of women in this world today who do fast, however not for religious reasons or beliefs.

They fast so they look like the stick insect models that walk the catwalks of the world and appear in numerous glossy magazines looking anorexic.

I only had to fast for around fifteen hours though. Not week after week like the thousands of women whose dream it is to have a body like their idols.

What crap. I prefer my women (that's only Sarah of course) to have some curves on them.

I bet if you asked the general public, most of them would say they like a bit of meat on their partners.

Sarah has to like it or lump it as far as my body is concerned. Yes there is one part of my body, namely my gut, that is podgy, but I don't care.

Of course I'd like to have a six-pack, but this blooming exercise lark is hard work. Although I will admit that I do some exercise each day. You want to see my remote control finger. It's toned, it's muscular and there's not a wrinkle on it!

Lots of people have commented that it's the best remote control finger they have ever seen. I did send a photo of it once to a men's health magazine, however I'm still waiting to hear back from them.

All I ever see in the health magazines are six-packs, bulging biceps and fit tanned bodies of good-looking men. How many men do you see like this when you go down the local for a pint? None, because they are stuck in the gym 24 hours a day making sure their triceps look good in the mirror. That life is definitely not for me thanks. Okay, so I am jealous. I admit it. I'd love to have a six-pack, eat healthy food everyday and have a ridiculously skinny bird bouncing on my bollocks all night long. But I can't. I'm married, work full time and have two kids who demand my attention when I get home. It's bloody impossible to lead the dream lifestyle. I haven't got time and I can't afford it.

However, it's taken me a long time to tone up my remote control finger and I think it's high time the magazines showed it. I'm still waiting to hear back as I write my story and this is seven years on! I suppose the seven year wait does send out the message that they are not interested, however I'm still optimistic that one day a magazine will devote its entire centre spread on how to achieve the perfect remote control finger. Anyway it's their loss.

Right, back to my stomach. I've got a podgy gut because I eat what I want to eat. However, in today's society you can't eat anything without the bloody health brigade getting on your case and saying it's bad for you. The way they carry on means you can't eat anything without it leading to cancer, heart disease, high cholesterol, etc etc. The dozy health brigade preach their message of eat this and don't eat that. The trouble is they tell us that nearly every type of food in existence is bad for you in some form or another. Take this as an example. One week they say eggs are good for you and then the next they are bad and can lead to high cholesterol. So what the hell can we eat then without us suffering an early death? I'll tell you what. Eat what the hell you want and don't listen to these tossers.

Unfortunately, some people do listen to these twats and they end up eating very little and becoming ill and all because they avoid the foods that are supposedly bad for you. Some message the health brigade preaches!

I say enjoy your food. When your time's up your time's up. I've seen too many fitness fanatics drop down dead in the prime of their life. I'm not saying exercising and eating healthily is wrong, because I've done it in the past myself (when I was single and had time and money). In moderation it's fine, but letting it rule your life is a bit extreme in my opinion.

Right back to my story. Where was I? Oh yes, the fasting. I tried to get rid of my hunger pangs by keeping myself busy. I decided I would read until the time came for my op. I read the daily newspaper word for word and then decided to visit the hospital shop to buy another magazine. I'd already read all the other ones Sarah had left me. I was supposed to be reading my financial adviser course notes, but to be honest with you they were boring. I much preferred reading about real life stories, rather than how to persuade a rich divorcee to part with a hundred grand.

I entered the hospital shop and was greeted by hundreds upon hundreds of chocolate bars. I heard a Double Decker say, "Eat me," and then a Twix shout, "I'll fill you up."

"Be strong man," I thought to myself. If I eat something then I've buggered up my operation and I would have to wait another day.

No way. I resisted the treats on offer, gave them the

middle finger and made my way to the magazine rack.

My eyes scanned the entire contents. What did I fancy reading about today? Every magazine I looked at I'd already read. Over the past day or so I'd read about affairs, murders, revenge, fitness, health and of course the problem pages.

Only this morning I'd learnt of some bloke who arrived home early from work and found his missus in bed with two other women. He'd written in to Dear Barbara for advice. She waffled on about trust, commitment and forgiveness. What utter shit! If I were the agony aunt my reply would have been as follows:

"Here's what you do my friend. Stop moaning, strip off and get in there you lucky bastard and service all three women with your love truncheon."

Some men just don't know when they've got a good thing going!

One magazine caught my eye. Horse and Hound. It must be about fox hunting I thought. Now I like a good debate and surely this magazine would give me a non-biased account of the pros and cons of fox hunting.

I didn't even have a quick flick through it. I just brought it based on the name alone. An intellectual read before I have my op. Just what the Doctor ordered.

I sat down on my bed and engaged my brain ready for some hard reading and debating. I opened the first page and then turned to the next one. I turned some more pages until I came to the end. Not a fox hunting debate in sight. It was all about horse riding and show jumping. If I wanted a cheap pair of jodhpurs then this was the right mag. However I didn't. They don't make them big enough for my thighs. This magazine wasn't for me after all.

Mind you, there was one interesting article about a pair of 18-year-old identical twins and their horses. Two stunning brunettes with two mighty stallions between their legs, two pairs of tight jodhpurs and two pairs of black knee high boots. This was more like it. I didn't read the article though; I just looked at the pictures instead.

As I finished this truly inspiring article a nurse and a porter were walking towards me.

Surely they can't be coming to get me. It's only 11.30am and I was due in around one o'clock.

The bloke next to me was due in before me to sort out his pissing. He told me that he was in agony every time he went and that he couldn't stop going. He went nearly every five minutes or so. Poor sod. Whilst he's in agony he can't stop peeing. Yet you can bet your bottom dollar that when he is fixed he won't be able to pee for love nor money. Another example of how life is a bitch.

My heart pounded, my mouth was dry and loads of little butterflies merrily flapped their wings in my stomach as the nurse and porter inched ever closer.

Yes I wanted the op to be done and dusted. I wanted to get rid of those awful feelings of nervousness and also I was starving and fancied a chip buttie.

Trouble is, this waiting around lark screws me up and my mind starts to think negatively. What if I don't pull through the op? I've heard of many people not pulling through because their bodies have an adverse reaction to the anaesthetic. Christ, what with the state of my body, I might as well give up now. This was my first operation and I was crapping myself.

The only way I can describe what I was feeling was this; I counted down every minute until my operation, not knowing whether I would see my wife and kids again.

I would picture Leah and Charlie when they were older. Charlie was having driving lessons and Leah would be dating. All the normal things you do when you are over 17 years of age. Although in this modern world, some kids as young as ten go joyriding and some girls get pregnant at eleven. Utter madness.

I pictured Charlie running into the house in utter jubilation, having passed his driving test. Sarah threw her arms around him and gave him a big hug. I didn't hug him though.

I saw Leah bringing home her first proper boyfriend and introducing him to Sarah and Charlie. I didn't meet him though. Why wasn't I involved in these things? Because I wasn't there.

I was dead and I couldn't share in these momentous occasions with them. I want to be able to help Charlie wash his new car every Sunday. I want to check out Leah's boyfriend and make sure he is good enough for her. I want to pick her up from right outside the nightclub doors at 10 o'clock, even though she is 19 years old. However, these simple pleasures may not happen if I don't pull through the operation.

This hurt like hell. I tried to get rid of these images and feelings by thinking of happier times, but it was no use. They were stuck in my head. They just wouldn't budge.

Granted, the likelihood of dying under the knife was minimal, but it could happen. This little seed of doubt was now planted firmly in my brain. However, there was one small crumb of comfort. I suppose if I don't make it, at least I'll get to see Mum and Dad again. Providing I'm allowed into heaven. Bloody hell, I wish I never pulled the legs off all them Daddy Long Legs in my youth. Does harming God's creatures mean an instant passage to hell? Surely not. Saying words like fuck, shit and bastard. Now that would mean no entry into heaven. Oh dear. That means you, the reader, are now destined for hell because you just said these words in your mind or read them out loud. Oh well. At least hell has got a nice climate and the heating bills are low. Okay, so I've said these words as well. Will I see you there? No way. Over the next few pages you will read about my cunning plan to gain entry into heaven. It's a cracker!

The nurse and porter were now only yards away. Christ, I'm not ready for this. Please don't take me. Part of me cries out, "Get it over with," and the other part cries out, "I'm shitting myself, I don't want to die!"

Deep down I hoped they had come for the bloke in the next bed. I was bloody bricking it. I turned away, hoping that if I didn't make eye contact then they wouldn't see me.

Then I heard the words, "Right Mr Barrett, it's time for your operation."

Thank God for that. It wasn't my turn after all. I got myself in such a state as well. Silly twat. The relief was paramount. Thank God, thank Allah, thank Buddha.

Those awful images immediately left my head and I could relax again. Well, for one and a half hours at least.

"Good luck," I shouted to him as he was wheeled away by the porter.

"Cheers," he replied nervously.

"You will be next Mr Couchman," said the nurse.

Thanks darling. All those awful images and fears immediately came back into my mind upon her finishing her sentence. So much for relaxing for the next hour and a half!

I suppose I now know that when the nurse and porter next perform their dreaded walk again, then it'll be my turn.

I felt sick and the insides of my stomach were doing somersaults.

I wish them pesky butterflies would piss off and fly into someone else's gut. I knew what was needed. Yes a pre-op dump. I've never done a pre-op dump before, mainly because I've never had an op before. I've done pre-match dumps before footie matches and I've done pre-exam dumps at school and at work. Christ, I've even done a pre-honeymoon night dump. I know they've all worked before to get rid of any butterflies I had, although the honeymoon dump did kill the romance somewhat.

Just as Sarah lay on the bed to reveal her sexy black lingerie, I felt myself touching cloth. I couldn't help it, I was nervous. Sarah said she'd never heard of anyone using the smell of rotting cabbage and sprouts as an aphrodisiac before. There's always a first time for everything.

I made my way towards the hospital bog to see if the pre-op dump would do the trick.

Fifteen minutes later I came out of the bog feeling a stone lighter. It had worked. Hurrah!

All my butterflies had flapped off down the u-bend and were halfway across the English Channel by now.

The only downside was a sore arse had replaced my butterflies. Mind you, you can't have it all I guess!

My sore arse had only been created by the hospital toilet paper. Jesus, that stuff is hard. It's like wiping your arse with sandpaper. And it looks like the tracing paper stuff we used to use at school. It's crap. It doesn't absorb anything; instead it just spreads it around even more. Why oh why can't the NHS invest in some quilted bog roll?

Do the surgeons really want to see a pile of shit caked around my buttocks? No they don't. If anyone from the NHS is reading this, I plea from my heart, get some Charmin in your bogs.

If it's good enough for the bears in the advert, then it's good enough for human beings.

I left the bog and made my way back to my bed, whilst walking like John Wayne.

I felt okay after my dump, but I still had around an hour to wait till my op and I didn't really want to think of dying again. What shall I do to kill an hour of time? Of course. I put on the radio headphones and listened to that awful DJ wannabe on Hospital FM. Please play Donny Osmond, I want a kip. This will take my mind off the op and stop those negative images returning.

I drifted off into a deep sleep as Donny belted out, "And they call it puppy love…………"

I was awoken by the nurse shaking my body.

"It's your turn now Mr Couchman,"she said.

I looked at the clock on the wall. Bloody hell it's 1.45pm.

"You're running late," I said.
"I know, apologies for that. A patient had difficulty breathing during their op and it was touch and go for a while," she explained.

Stone me love, did you have to tell me all the details. This fills me with complete confidence, not.

My heart pounds, my mouth resembles a dried out oasis and them sodding butterflies have re-appeared. The images of me not being around in the future resurface again. Shit.

This is it. No turning back now.

"Good luck," the old duffers all shouted.

"Be strong, show them you've got balls," said one of the old gits.

Is he taking the piss? Then it hit me. I might only have the singular of balls when I come out of my operation. I can't keep my legs crossed forever.

I hadn't thought about this all morning. My mind had quite rightly been pre-occupied with thoughts about Sarah, Leah and Charlie.

However, now I needed a bit of alone time with my bollocks. This could be the last time I ever have two. Christ, I might only have about five minutes left to spend with my two close friends. Sorry my dear wife and kids. I've thought about you lots this morning but I've got to stop thinking about you now. My thoughts are needed elsewhere. This is an emergency.

As I was being wheeled through the corridors I tried to think of a really good send off for my right bollock, just in case.

I couldn't have a wank to relieve the poor chap before he leaves the safety of my sack. No, too many people around. What could I do?

There was only one thing I could do. Have a rummage down below. No one will see me as I've got a sheet over me.

I put my hands down below and affectionately played with my bollocks. A tear appeared in my eye. Don't well up you soppy sod. Your bollocks wouldn't want to see you cry. Shape up man, hold it together.

I thought about asking the nurse if she fancied joining in this historical moment, but she was too busy chatting to the porter about last night's episode of Eastenders. There's me contemplating life with one bollock and they're more interested in whether Frank and Pat are getting back together.

Finally, after being wheeled through more corridors than the Crystal Maze, we arrived at theatre. I brought a Joseph And His Amazing Technicolor Dreamcoat programme (eight sodding quid), a bottle of fizzy water and some dolly mixtures. I was ready for the show.

The porter pushed me through the double doors and the anaesthetist greeted me.

"Good afternoon Mr Couchman," he said, "Welcome to theatre."

"Is this Joseph show any good," I asked him?

He just laughed and said, "The old ones are the best!"

I was only trying to break the ice and put myself at ease.

Next to me I could see a silver tray and on it were displayed various needles ranging from very small to outrageously long.

"Why all the different sizes?" I thought to myself.

Then it struck me. Of course, the bigger you are as a person the more anaesthetic you need. It's calculated on a dosage to weight ratio.

Small people like Ronnie Corbett or the Oompa Loompas from Charlie and the Chocolate Factory have the small needles, because they don't need as much anaesthetic. The big bastards, like Jabba the Hutt or a sumo wrestler, need more anaesthetic so they have the big needles. Simple really.

Holy shit! That means I'm going to get the biggest needle going. I wish I had stuck to my Ryvita and bran flakes diet. True, I spent more on Charmin and Toilet Duck because I was so regular, but at least I would've been guaranteed a teeny weenie needle. Oh well, I can't do anything about it now.

"Let's get on with it then Mr Couchman," the anaesthetist said. "I'm going to give you the anaesthetic and then I want you to close your eyes and count backwards from five."

"Only from five?" I replied very surprised.

"Yes from five. I guarantee you'll be in a deep sleep before you reach number one," he said with confidence.

"Must be good stuff then," I added.

"The best Mr Couchman," he said with pride.

Now, remember my earlier myth of the bigger you are the longer the needle you get. Well this was blown completely out of the window.

There are no long needles. Instead they use a candular. This is basically a medical instrument that is placed upon the back on your hand and fastened with tape. A very small needle on the end of the candular is then directed into the vein on the back of your hand. A tube is then connected to it and the anaesthetic is pumped into the bloodstream via the tube. Simple and not a monster needle in sight.

"A tiny prick Mr Couchman," he said as he inserted the candular into my vein.

"Yes I have Doc," I said embarrassingly. " Does the size of my nob affect the dosage then?" He didn't answer.

What I wanted to know was this. Why have all them bloody long needles on display? It doesn't matter what size you are, because the anaesthetist uses a candular every time.

I reckon it's for dramatic effect. I've seen Casualty and Holby City. I've seen the long scalpel, the 12-inch needle and the Black and Decker drill all neatly laid out on the silver tray. However, I've never seen an episode yet where they are used. They are placed on the tray to make the scene seem more dramatic.

Tell a lie, there was an episode of Casualty where the Black and Decker drill was used. A workman had to put up a new notice board in A&E!

I closed my eyes and the anaesthetist drew back the

curtain to see for certain…Wait a minute. I know these words.

"Have a nice dream," he said.
"What shall I dream," I asked.

"Oh, any dream will do," he replied.

Bloody hell. They were showing Joseph after all. I didn't want to miss it, but the anaesthetic that was pumped into my vein started to take effect immediately. 5,4,3…

That's all I can remember. I tried desperately to prove all the medical experts wrong and get to number one. However, it wasn't to be.

As the anaesthetist said,

"It's the best."

Too right it's the best! I couldn't believe how quick it had worked on me.

I mean, there's a lot of mass that the anaesthetic had to get round; yet I only got to number three. I was fairly disappointed in myself. And I missed the bloody show.

Apparently the record in the hospital for counting backwards, whilst the anaesthetic is pumped in, is minus 150. What a star!

I later found out that when the patient in question reached minus 140, the anaesthetist realised the needle hadn't gone into the vein properly, therefore rendering the anaesthetic useless. Kind of mucks up the record I suppose. I think it should still stand. After all it wasn't the patient's fault was it?

Right where was I. Oh yes 5,4,3 …

The next thing I remember was hearing someone

calling "Darren, Darren?"

I slowly opened my eyes and I felt really spaced out. The first thing I saw was a really bright light above my head.

The call came again, "Darren, Darren?"

I turned my head slowly towards the calls. I saw a young blonde women leaning over me. Her boobs were nearly touching me. Crikey, they were like two watermelons trying to escape from a shopping bag. I was fairly drowsy at this point, however the boobs did their best to awaken me properly.

"Darren, Darren, are you with us?" the young lady said.

She then started to rub my brow with her gentle hands and then ran them through my hair.

"I'm bloody dead," I thought. I must be. I didn't make it through the op.

Feeling spaced out, no pain, the bright light and the gorgeous young lady stroking my brow whilst her two great melons swayed to and fro. I must be in heaven. This must be what heaven is like and the best bit of all is God is a woman with huge tits. Nice. I always had a feeling God was a Woman. Look at the facts.

Us men got the raw end of the deal when it came to dishing out the private parts. I mean, when was the last time you heard a woman say,

"Blimey, your cock is the best looking thing I have ever seen."

I've never heard these words and I'm sure there are countless men out there in the same boat as me.

Yet when it comes to the vagina, it's a different matter altogether. They are a work of art and bloody good-looking things too. They are also magical. A few strokes of the razor and hey presto. They turn into something even more beautiful!

That's why I have always felt God is a lady. She looks after her own and makes sure us blokes suffer. Of course the argument will carry on for evermore. However, I'm confident lots of blokes will agree with my theory. Right, back to the female with the large melons.

"Darren, you've had your op and you are now in the recovery room," said the young women. "It all went well. How do you feel?"

I could just about nod my head and say, "Okay." I was still fairly out of it, but then I realised I was alive and wasn't in heaven. Relief spread throughout my entire body, although I was looking forward to seeing Mum and Dad again. Oh, and of course, playing with God's huge knockers.

I'm alive and I'm grateful. I've got my own family now. They need me and I need them. I can't leave them now. I've got so much I want to do with them all. There'll be plenty of time when I die to see Mum and Dad again. I'm sure they understand.

Mind you, when I do die, I bloody hope heaven is like what I described earlier. I won't be afraid of death at all.

I'll be on my deathbed and the nurse will be saying, "Hold on Mr Couchman, your family will be here very shortly."

"Well can they get a move on?" I reply. "Only there's a queue building up to play with God's tits."

I'd better explain that the bright light I saw was the hospital light on the ceiling and not the bright light you supposedly see when you are dying.

I wasn't in pain because the anaesthetic was still in

my body and it was also making me drowsy as well.

And it wasn't God with huge tits, it was a pretty young nurse called Louise.

However, I've started praying every night since. "Please God may you be a women who walks around heaven in your Sloggi sports bra and thong?" I can only hope.

"But you won't get into heaven because of all your swearing," I hear you cry. True. But this is the cunning plan I mentioned earlier. All this praying should outweigh all the times I've sworn and at least guarantee me an interview with God. I fucking hope so!

I was taken back to the ward around thirty minutes later. The Doctors and nurses were happy with my vital stats, like my blood pressure, pulse rate, etc. They were also happy that my op had all gone to plan.

I was still fairly drowsy and tired when I got back to the ward. All I wanted to do was sleep. A nurse made me drink some water, as I hadn't had a drink for some time. I can't tell you how good that felt, as my mouth was as dry as a retired hooker's fanny.

The nurse said the Doctor would come and see me in a couple of hours to have a chat about the operation and to discuss the next steps.

I was very sleepy now and I drifted off into a deep sleep.

It wasn't until later when Sarah and my brother James visited me that I didn't even give a thought about whether I had two bollocks or one. I was tired, so tired, that it just consumed my whole body and took over.

James woke me up. That little sleep hadn't helped in anyway reduce my tiredness.

I could just about make out what they were saying.

"How are you feeling?" Sarah asked.

"Bloody tired," I replied.

I know they had come to see me and for that I was grateful, but I just couldn't stop my eyelids from closing every couple of seconds.

"Get some rest," Sarah answered.

"Stop asking me bloody questions then!" I said to myself.

However, bruv had to ask one more. It turned out to be a cracker of a question.

"How many bollocks you got now then bruv?" he asked.

It was this question that made me realise that I didn't even know the answer. Had one of my close mates gone forever? All I could think of after my op was to sleep. Suddenly I became more alert. This was something I needed to know and quick. This was the most important question in the world right now.
Fuck the questions like,

"How do we achieve world peace?" and "How do we stop global warming?"

I just wanted to know how many bollocks I had left.

Chapter 5
One Lump or Two?

I didn't know the answer to my brother's question.

"I've been asleep since the op and it didn't even occur to me to ask," I said now very concerned.

The Doctor would be another good hour and I couldn't wait this long. The suspense was killing me and Sarah and James were just as eager to find out.

James more so because he had a bet with the old boy opposite that I would still have two left.

It was time to open my NHS gown and have a feel.

James pulled the curtains around us all. The anticipation was so high; it was like waiting for the FA Cup draw to be made.

I pulled the sheet over me, as I didn't want bruv looking at my nob. We may be identical twins, but I'm pretty sure we don't have identical cocks.

We've always been competitive and I don't want to give him any bragging rights over my Walnut Whip.

I opened my gown and slowly my hand reached down towards my sack.

I then pulled my hand up quickly as though I had a sodding piranha down my pants, ready to bite my fingers off.

"I can't do it," I said scared. "I'll wait for the Doctor."

"No way bruv," James replied, "I've got a fiver riding on this. Feel your bollocks now!"

I took a deep breath and put my hand down below. I fiddled around for about five seconds and I knew straightaway the outcome.

"You've lost your bet," I said to James, whilst letting out a huge sigh.

"Shit," he shouted angrily.

He then realised the full extent of what I had just said.

"Jesus bruv, I'm sorry about your bollock," he added.

Sarah sat down in the chair and grabbed my hand.

"Remember what the surgeon told you. You can still lead a perfectly normal life with one," Sarah said trying to reassure me.
"But what about the sex?" I asked Sarah.

"Sex," Sarah replied all puzzled. "Well I assume your testicle is a male."

"No not the sex of my testicle you daft moo. You know. Our sex life. That thing we do once a year on my birthday," I said sarcastically. "What if I can't perform properly?"

"You can't perform now," Sarah laughed. "So I wouldn't worry about it."

Thanks for making me feel great and on top of the

world dear wife.

"I'm only joking," she continued. "You'll be fine with one. In fact you might even try harder with just the one, you never know."

Sarah then crossed her fingers, looked up towards the ceiling and mouthed,

"Please God let him try harder. Then I might stay awake!"

My head was spinning and I felt sick. It had hit me like a ten tonne brick. Yes I had laughed with my mate weeks earlier up in Leeds when he was taking the piss and telling jokes about having one bollock. However, back then I had two and there was still the small chance I wouldn't lose it. Also, as I said earlier, I'd reassured myself that I would wake up with two. Bugger.

This was reality now. It had happened and there was fuck all I could do about it. My poor redundant bollock all on his own. He did have the tumour for company, although tumours are not known to socialise very well. He's probably floating around in some specimen jar, missing his other buddy. I bet he's really lonely and scared. What was to become of him?

Yes he was to be sent off to the lab for my results to see if the tumour was cancerous or not, but what about after that?

What does the NHS do with useless bollocks? Throw them in the bin? Perhaps even re-cycle them? They might put the specimen jar containing my bollock in a cupboard and close the doors forever. The cupboard would be marked "useless testicles." Perhaps they burn them and play the song "Great Balls of Fire" as a nice send off. I don't know. To be honest I didn't want to know.

I like to think that my bollock was put to good use, perhaps being used to show student Doctors what a bollock with a tumour looks like. Or best of all placed in a pickled jar with lots of other bollocks and put on the surgeon's shelf, proudly looking out across his office. My bollock would have a new family and he could enjoy his early retirement in peace.

However, what about the one he had left behind? Poor bastard. There's nothing worse than being on your own and being Billy no mates.

I decided at this point that my solitary bollock would receive the utmost love and affection from myself and hopefully Sarah as well. Christ, I didn't want my only bollock to commit suicide from depression.

I gently cupped him in my hands and told him, "You are my one and only ball and one hell of a special testicle." Jesus, I'm a poet. I bet Wordsworth never wrote a poem about a bollock, as he wandered lonely like a cloud.

My bollock was going to need a lot of loving now it would be doing the work of two. Hard times lie ahead for you my friend, but with courage and strength and with a lot of help from Daddy's wrists, you can achieve anything you want.

I had to be strong also. The clock can't be turned back. As I said earlier I'm a firm believer in fate. Things happen for a reason. God (the bitch) has meant for me to have one bollock and there must be a really good reason for doing so. I couldn't think of a good reason at the time, however I prayed that something good would come out of this terrible mess and would show itself in the future. Only time would tell.

"I'm okay," I said to Sarah and James. "I've got to accept I've only got one bollock now. It's going to be hard but I'll get used to it."

"Nice one," Sarah said relieved. "We'll not let this affect our lives and ruin them. Lets be positive. We've got to make sure that only good can come out of this situation." Her fingers were still crossed and again she looked skywards and prayed. However, she could see that her regular conversations with the almighty were upsetting me. She continued,

"Look, I was mucking about earlier when I said about you trying harder. Having one will make no difference to our sex life. Nothing will change."

Well apart from the fact that you'll only have one bollock slapping against the backs of your thighs in the future.

Might make a nice change though and it'll probably have a different sound to it. Less noisy with one. See, straightaway I was thinking positively about only having one bollock. A smile appeared on my face.

"What you grinning at?" Sarah asked.

"Nothing," I replied. "I'm going to have fun with my solitary friend," I thought to myself.

I felt relieved. I had accepted my new situation fairly quickly and I felt very proud of how I had dealt with such a blow. Sod it I thought. Having one bollock isn't the end of the world; it's the start of a new era. Okay, so the only positive thing I had thought of was that sex might sound different with one bollock. Surely this isn't the reason why God has taken one of my bollocks. No it can't be. There's got to be a bigger reason than this. I was confident that a lot more positives would show themselves and soon I would find out the real reason why God nicked my bollock. I just hope she hadn't run out of ping-pong balls whilst playing table tennis and decided my testicle would be an ideal replacement. Now that would be a kick in the bollock! Losing my testicle just so God could be crowned ping-pong champion of heaven.

In that instant I didn't feel tired or drowsy anymore. I felt alive and on top of the world. Yes I know it's probably weird to get over something like this so quickly, but I was still the same Darren. Nothing's changed apart from the fact that I'm six pounds lighter in my never regions and that sex may well be less noisy. Oh, and the fact that I might have cancer. Then again I might not. I'll deal with that when I get my results in a couple of weeks.

Time had flown by whilst I was contemplating life with one bollock.

The Doctor had arrived for his chat.

Sarah and James went to the canteen to get a drink and I was left alone with the Doctor and a nurse.

He got the pleasantries out of the way first and then he asked me to produce my package for inspection.

"The operation went really well Mr Couchman, however I'm afraid we had to remove your right testicle," Doc said. "The tumour was very large and had engulfed your testicle. I'm very sorry."

At this point I could've pretended I didn't know and wailed and wept like an Oscar winner, but I didn't.

"I know Doc, I've had a feel," I replied. "But I'm okay about it all."

"That's good," said Doc. "I'm glad you're thinking positively. Remember, your life will in no way be affected by this."

"Oh it will," I answered. "This is life changing, but for the better." I was grinning like a prostitute who'd been given the all clear at the clinic.

"Right," he said looking confused. He changed the

subject quickly.

"Let's have a look at your wound and make sure it's all in order shall we?" he added.

I sat up, trying to have a butchers at what the wound looked like and how big my scar may be. I want it to be a big one. Then I can lie and tell everyone about the time I fought a crocodile and won.

I looked down and my world collapsed. The bastards! They had only gone and shaved half my pubes off. Just the right side. Bloody hell it looked weird. Why didn't they go the whole hog and shave the lot off? At least then it would've looked more in proportion. They didn't tell me this when they were briefing me about my op.

It has only gone and ruined my woman's vagina trick. I can't push my tackle between my legs now and pretend to be a lady. I've never seen a fanny half shaved and half hairy before. Hold on though. Variety is the spice of life. This new look could catch on.

Single women everywhere could adopt this look and it would cater for both sides of the fanny market. Some men like it shaved and some prefer a great big wiry bush. I think I'll have to patent this idea and get a copyright on it before some bird from Brazil invents it. I'll call it "The multi-purpose minge."

"All looks fine to me Mr Couchman," Doc said.

"I'm starting to feel some pain now Doc," I replied.
"Most probably," he answered. "The anaesthetic will be wearing off now. The nurse will get you some strong painkillers to help with the pain."

"Cheers Doc," I said with my face now grimacing.

"Rest up now Mr Couchman and if all's going to plan

you can go home tomorrow," Doc added.

That's what I wanted to hear. Get home and get back to normal. I could read up on my boring course notes and be ready to resume my training as a financial adviser the following Monday. Sounds realistic. Christ, I've only had a bollock removed, not a leg!

The Doctor said he would come and see me again tomorrow and if the pain gets worse, I'm to ask the nurse for some painkillers. Sounds easy enough.

Sarah and James returned from the canteen. James gave the old boy opposite his five pounds winnings from the bet. The old git immediately got out of his bed and announced he was going to the hospital shop to buy a mag entitled "Saga Sally does Skegness."

I explained to them everything the Doctor had told me and that hopefully I would be home tomorrow.

"That's great!" Sarah announced.

"You'll have to look after me and wait on me for the rest of the week though. Doctor's orders," I said, lying through my back teeth.

"So what's new?" she replied sarcastically.

By now the pain across my groin, where the incision had been made, was getting worse.

Every time I moved I was in agony. I just couldn't get comfortable. It felt like someone was tugging hard on my groin from the inside. A bloody weird feeling, but also a bloody painful one.

Thirty minutes later it was unbearable. Tears were welling up in my eyes and it felt like vinegar was being poured over my wound. I've never felt pain like it before.

Well, apart from the time when England lost to Germany on penalties in the 1990 world cup and most Saturdays when Spurs cock up.

I tried to be a man. Well, as best I could, seeing as I only had one bollock now and half a set of pubes. I gritted my teeth and tried to put up with the pain. I don't need painkillers. I'm going to be a hero. Sarah needs a hero, she's been holding out for a hero till the end of the night. I've got to be strong and I've got to be larger than life.

I pictured myself running from a burning building clutching a baby or diving into the raging sea in my red swim shorts to rescue a drowning kiddie, whilst David Hasselhoff watched on in awe.

It was no use though. The pain wouldn't go, no matter how many times I rescued kids from disaster and cats from trees.

Time to swallow my pride and swallow some painkillers.

James went and asked the nurse for some. He said it was probably best if he went as he could clearly see I wasn't up to walking. What a generous nature he has. Of course it's nothing to do with the fact that the nurse was gorgeous and he wanted a rectal examination!

I swallowed the tablets and prayed they would get to work fast.

Within about fifteen minutes they had kicked in and the pain started to subside. Not completely, although now it was bearable.

The only problem was they were so bloody strong they made me drowsy. I tell you what, it's a good job I wasn't going to drive or operate machinery that day. That's how drowsy I felt. Whilst I'm on this subject, see if you can make this out:

On children's pain relief medicines it states that one of the possible side effects is drowsiness. Some years ago I came across a leading brand of children's medicine that stated, "If you become drowsy, please ensure you do not drive or operate machinery." What the hell are they on about? When did you last see an eight year old get into his or her Mondeo and drive off to the factory to do a 12-hour shift on his or her industrial lathe? I swear to you I've seen this on several leading brands, although I think most of them have now changed their wording. Mind you, I think they need to put these words back on. Some young kids do drive for a living. It's called joyriding. And some young kids operate machinery. They're called guns.

Anyway, I started to doze off and Sarah and James agreed it would be best if they went and let me get some valuable rest.

We said our goodbyes and Sarah said she would visit again tomorrow.

Just as I closed my eyes my mate from the course and his girlfriend turned up bearing grapes and Lucozade.

I was really knackered, but they had made the effort to come and see me. I couldn't go asleep now. How rude would that look?

They said they wouldn't stay long as they could see I looked tired. Too bloody right.

I confidently told my mate that I would be okay for next Monday and would be travelling up to Leeds as planned.

He didn't seem to share my enthusiasm and said to see how I felt in a few days. However, I was adamant I would be going.

We chatted away as best I could, in between my eyelids closing and my head dropping.

However, true to their word they buggered off after half an hour. I told him I would give him a call that weekend to sort out the travel arrangements to Leeds.

At last I could get some sleep.

The painkillers were still working and I nestled my head snugly on my pillow. I pulled up the sheet and blanket and drifted off to Baywatch where the Hoff

Meister and me were discussing the pros and cons of tit jobs.

What a dream. I was just about to inspect a stunning brunette's big knockers when I heard a voice say,

"Dinner's ready, are you having some?"

I slowly opened my eyes to see the catering lady with her large trolley of delights. The ward was filled with a lovely smell of home cooking and baked bread. Oh all right, the ward still stank of disinfectant and piss. Not even the smell of fine cuisine could mask that awful aroma.

I was starving, seeing as I hadn't eaten for hours. The nurse had offered me toast after my op, but I didn't fancy anything then. Why do we always get offered toast? Why can't the nurses drum up a nice pie and mash with lots of gravy?

"Yeah, I'll have some please," I said to the catering lady. "What have you got?"

"Meatballs," she replied.

Bloody marvellous I thought. Is she taking the piss? Why don't you just serve up my redundant bollock in spaghetti sauce and *really* rub it in.

"Fine, I'll have the meatballs," I said. "But if you give me two or less meatballs I'll burn your trolley."

"Tea or coffee?" she then asked.

"Tea please with milk and sugar," I replied.

"One lump or two?" she said.

Right, that was one step too far. I still can't believe I didn't do time for setting fire to one hundred meatballs and four trays of chips. I pleaded post-op trauma and they felt sorry for me I reckon.

About an hour later I needed a pee. I hadn't been since the op and I was desperate.

Listening to the catering lady pouring out endless cups of tea didn't help. There's something about flowing liquids, particularly water, that makes me want to pee. Even a dripping tap sets me off. Imagine if I visited Niagara Falls? I'd have to wear a Tena lady to absorb all my piss.

Right, shall I buzz for assistance so the nurse can help me do a piss, or shall I try to go on my own?

I've never needed help before so why should I start now. Besides, I'm a hero. I slowly turned my feet round towards the side of my bed. I had some slight pain, but I felt okay. The painkillers were still doing their job. I stood up, my first time since the op. I hope my legs still work. They did.

Now normally I'd run or take big strides towards the bog when I'm desperate, but in this instance I couldn't. I could only shuffle and take small pigeon steps, because I was sore where the incision had been made. However, I was determined to make it to the bog and not fall short and end up pissing on the ward floor. E.T.A to the bog was five minutes I reckoned, judging by the distance and the size of my steps. Slowly I edged ever forwards towards my target.

I did it in six minutes and not my original target of five. This was only because some old duffer cut me up in his Zimmer frame and I spent one minute telling the old sod that if he ever did that again I would melt down his Zimmer, make it into an iron poker and then shove it in his japs eye.

I still felt proud having made it to the bog though. Like reaching the North Pole, scaling Everest, or landing on the moon. I planted the English flag in the shower cubicle to show every man that I did it and to ensure the memory of my epic trek to the khazi lives on.

I did my pee (a bloody long one too) and as I looked down I was again reminded that I only had half a set of pubes. Christ, the shaven area was now really itchy and sore. How women have a kojak down below is beyond me.

It was on my journey back from the North Bog to the South Bed that I didn't feel right. I felt sick and the room started spinning. I felt really dizzy. I tried to control my balance, but it was no use. Down I came crashing, onto my hands and knees. Christ that hurt. Nurses came running from every direction to help me.

"What are you doing out of bed Mr Couchman?" a nurse asked.

"I needed a pee," I replied.

"Mr Couchman," she said sternly, "You're still going to be dizzy because of the anaesthetic and the strong painkillers. It's still in your system. Why didn't you buzz for help?"

"You're very busy," I said, "And besides, I didn't want to take up three nurses just to hold my nob and guide my pee into the pan."

The nurse chuckled and said,

"We both know that it wouldn't take three nurses now would it Mr Couchman?"

Bloody hell, all the nurses must have seen my nob or

read the Doctor's notes at some stage.

She continued, "Anyway, when I said buzz for help, I didn't mean we'd escort you to the toilet and then hold it. I'd have got you a bottle to pee in from the comfort of your own bed. Then you don't have to get up and fall over."

Bloody NHS. I bet if I went private the nurses would hold my nob and wipe my arse for me. What money can buy, eh?

The nurse helped me back into bed and I lay down and went to sleep. My epic journey had taken its toll.

That night was a bloody nightmare. I was in agony and no matter what way I slept the pain just got worse. Should I buzz for the nurses? I didn't want to. My hero status would disappear in an instant and one more buzz would mean hero to zero in a flash.

However, the pain was now the worse I had experienced since my op and tears were gushing out from my eyes. I had no choice but to buzz the nurses.

The nurse actually gave me some morphine as she could see how much pain I was in. This helped immensely and also sent me back off into a deep sleep. This morphine is bloody good stuff. Spaced out or what? I've seen it being used in war films on the hero who is badly injured. One shot of morphine into the thigh and the pain is gone. The hero would then relax and start gibbering on about someone writing to his wife should he die. It's all for dramatic effect I thought. However, now I had experienced the joys of morphine myself, I can hand on heart say it does kill the pain and it does leave you spaced out (depending on the dose of course).

Talking of morphine, did you know a lot of painkillers that you can buy over the counter at chemists contain codeine? This comes from the same family as heroin and *both* convert to morphine in the brain. Apparently there are tens of thousands of people in the UK who are dependant on these, many without even realising (well, the ones known about anyway), including one of my mates. The drug companies don't give any specific warnings about this in the leaflets, other than telling you not to take them for more than 3 days. That's really irresponsible, don't you think? Well I bloody think so.

The next morning came and went. I was feeling slightly better, but the pain and soreness were still evident.

The Doctor said that morning that if I was up to it, I could go home later on.

Now normally I'd be itching (like my pubes) to get home to see Leah and Charlie, as I hadn't seen them for a couple of days. Sarah and I thought it best they didn't visit and see me in this state, as it would upset them. Then they would start asking me lots of questions. Why followed by another why and so on. They were still young. They both knew I was in hospital, but not what for. They would've had trouble taking it all in at such tender ages. Christ, *I* struggled to take it all in and I was 27!

We both agreed they would be told when they were older. They would understand it more then. As far as they were concerned, Daddy was in hospital having a general MOT.

I made the decision to stay in for a couple more days. Yes I wanted to see the kids, but I also know that they like jumping on their Dad and having big cuddles and play fights.

Also I was still very sore and in considerable pain when the painkillers and morphine wore off. I would be a burden to Sarah in this state. She'd have to wait on me hand and foot. It was tempting though.

Also the bog at home was upstairs and although I'd trekked from South Bed to North Bog and back, I wasn't ready to scale Mount Khazi just yet.

My mind was made up. I'd rather go home knowing I could get around and do things for myself, rather than lay on the settee all day long watching my entire Only Fools and Horses DVD collection, followed by Blackadder Goes Forth. Looking back, I kind of regretted my decision to stay in. I then would have experienced another form of sheer bliss!

The next two days were very similar to the previous two, apart from the fact that I was getting better and the pain and soreness were slowly going away with each passing hour. And thank God, I could now go for a pee and a poo on my own. I got told off the previous night for trying to crap in the urine bottle. I didn't know. I thought it was used for number ones and number twos. Mind you, I did wonder at the time how my turd would fit into such a small opening. Luckily I had a dodgy belly from the meatballs and that problem never arose.

Breakfast, lunch and dinner arrived on the exact hour each day. The catering lady was her normal charming self. She now carried a fire extinguisher on her trolley because of the time I set fire to her meatballs and chips. At least she had a health and safety review after this. Did I get any thanks? No I didn't. I only highlighted the fact that if some angry patient set fire to her meatballs and chips, she would need a fire extinguisher nearby.

It's pretty boring staying in hospital because it's the same old routine every day. It's very mundane. There's only so many books and mags you can read before your brain is scrambled and crying out for a rest.

Yes there was the radio, but I still couldn't tune in Radio 1 or Five Live for the football and I'd had enough of listening to that smug twat on Hospital FM.

There was of course the TV in the ward that we all shared, but as I said earlier, I never got a look in with

Dads Army about.

To pass the time I'd try and guess all the nurses uniform and bra sizes. I'd then check back with them to see if I'd got them correct. However, once I'd done them all, that little game was over. So I then moved on to the wives of the old boys when they visited. Mind you with these ladies, if wasn't so much as guess the bra size, it was more like how far did their tits hang down. One old girl's tits were hanging so low she had to tuck them in her shoes!

The only time my boring day was broken up was when I had visitors.

Now hospital policy normally allows 2-3 visitors around each bed. I don't want to blow my own trumpet, but I've got lots of friends and also a huge family. 2-3 visitors. Bollock to that matron!

At one time I had eight visitors around my bed. Luckily matron turned a blind eye. She had grown fond of me. The day before was her birthday and I wished her a happy 30th. She was actually fifty but looked sixty, however I know how to treat a lady on her birthday and make her feel good. Plus I knew I would get lots of visitors and I needed her on my side. This had made her day and every time I pressed my buzzer for assistance, she would be there in an instant, helping me with whatever I needed. I even got three bed baths in one day! *And* my brother got his rectal examination.

I also had a guess that her uniform was a very petite size 10 and that her bra size was a compact 32C. In reality she was a dress size 18 and her bra was a 40DD. However, my estimates made her feel like a queen. I also said how nice she looked in her uniform (this was genuine as I like nurses uniforms). Not to wear myself you understand, I like the nurses to wear it.

All of this buttering up meant she was now firmly my bitch and would do what ever I wanted.

I could have as many visitors as I liked and no one

could say a word.

Two of the old duffers did moan though. However, matron soon told them to get over it, or she'd shove a thermometer up one of their arses and then use the same one on the next old moaner, but this time place it in his mouth. Good old matron.

I do remember one time, after having a large dose of morphine, that there were about twenty visitors around my bed. I remember it well, because I never realised that amongst this group of well-wishers I had a pink elephant, a unicorn and a fire-breathing dragon as mates. Weird or what.

Lots of family and friends came and went over the next two days. Each came bearing gifts, the same bloody gifts.

I reckon they all got together and agreed to buy grapes and Lucozade in bulk, just so they could get a fricking discount.

There's probably some little French guy in the South of France working 24 hours a day picking grapes, just so he can keep up with the demands of my family and friends. Mind you, it's about time the French did something in return for us Brits. We've waited nearly 68 years for them to return us a favour and yet they still shit on us (letting in loads of illegal immigrants through the tunnel for starters). Look, I don't dislike the French; the majority of them are fine. However, I tend to remember the bad occasions over the good ones. Before I even visited France I had an image in my mind of what the French people were like. A nation of people who only eat garlic, snails, frog legs and onions. A nation of people who wear berets on their heads and whose women have never come across a razor before. A nation of people who buckled easily when the Germans invaded. Now, before I am lynched and hung from the Eiffel Tower, I'd like to point out that these are not my own ideas of how I see the French. I've only got these pre-conceived misconceptions because that's what us English like to portray the French as. I've seen the little French man on his bike, wearing a beret and with half a tonne of onions hanging around his neck (although this is for show and attracts the tourists). I've been told that the French like to have garlic in every one of their meals, hence the smelly breath (yet us English seem to use garlic in everything as well). I've read the history books that say the French gave up too easily during the two world wars (what about the brave resistance fighters though in World War Two. Then there's the battle of Verdun during the First World War. What guts and courage the French displayed). And my mates have told me that all French girls don't shave their legs or their armpits (yet the ones I have come across have been as smooth as a baby's bottom). Blimey, I can't believe I'm sticking up for the French. It's all tosh, but that's the way us English like to see our French cousins and it will probably carry on like this for hundreds and hundreds of years. There has always been rivalry between our nations. The wars, the football and the rugby. It's all good banter. We like to take the piss out of the French and I'm sure they like doing it in return. It's the same with the Scots, the Irish and the Welsh. It's just a bit of fun. The trouble is that the few French people I have come across have left a bad taste in my mouth and this I don't forget.

Once when I was in Calais, my mates and I found a karaoke bar. I went up to sing and just because I chose Waterloo by Abba, all the frogs in the bar had a fit. They started muttering loads of crap in their French accents. Okay, so I took the piss a bit, but bloody hell, get over it Monsieur's. The battle of Waterloo was over 190 years ago.

Then there was the time I visited Euro Disney near Paris with Sarah and the kids. All day long I had made the effort to speak in French when I was ordering food. For example, I went into a burger bar and said the following,

"Deux Coca Cola for moi and trios burgers with fromage for mes missus and mes kiddies."

I thought I did bloody well and had hoped that, in return, the French would treat us all with respect. How sodding wrong could one be. The main Disney parade was on in thirty minutes. I gathered up the kids and Sarah and we made our way towards the parade route. We secured ourselves an excellent spot and in doing so, ensured that we wouldn't miss a thing. The kids were excited as the parade inched its way ever nearer to our position. Just as Mickey and Minnie walked past, about 100 French people started to push in and tried to take our spot. Wankers. Why didn't they show this type of aggression during the war? Maybe then it would have ended quicker (I'm just teasing). I stood my ground and elbowed a few in the ribs. I felt like Henry the Fifth (Henry V for all you historians) at the battle of Agincourt. Still the French came, but still I repelled every attack. One woman used her secret weapons and breathed all over me with her garlic breath and chucked onions at my head (again just having a laugh). I retaliated by pulling the hair under her arm. She sounded just like Chewbacca as she screamed out in pain. Mind you, she was bloody hairy (look I told you earlier, my mates told me about the under arm hair, so blame them, not me). I won the battle and ensured my kids saw the rest of the parade in peace. The French I encountered that day were bloody arrogant and rude. It's a shame really, because they spoil it for the rest of their nation and it gives France a bad reputation. Mind you, it happens here in England with the football hooligans. Lots of countries hate the English because of our reputation. The minority spoil it for the majority. Mind you, it probably happens in every country for some reason or another.

Now, you may well ask,

"Why was you in France in the first place if all you'd heard was bad things about them?"

Well, we'd only gone to Calais to stock up on stink bombs, nude playing cards and lots of plonk. And with Euro Disney, there was a cracking deal on offer. The beer and wine deals are the only good things in France. Actually not true. There are some cracking things the French can be proud of. Napoleon for starters, although he was defeated by the English at Waterloo. Joan of Arc, although I seem to remember she was burnt at the stake by the English. The French rugby team, although Jonny Wilkinson and Co did beat them in the 2003 World Cup semi-final. We then went on to win it. Arsenal Football Club. Yes I know it's an English club, but a Frenchman runs it and most of the players are French. Anyway, that's enough of the French. I've slagged them off enough.

I remember one visitor in particular who brightened up my day. One of my mates, Alan, turned up to see me. We were chatting away when all of a sudden his mobile phone rung. It was his missus and she was in town shopping. She was ringing to agree a pick up time from outside Wilkinsons.

"Jesus Al," I said, "You can't have your mobile on in here. It might interfere with the medical equipment."

"Course it won't," he answered, having blatantly ignored the twenty or so signs on the way in saying, " Please turn off your mobile phone."

"Anyway I need it on," he said. "I'm expecting some important texts."

"Well keep it hidden mate," I replied, "I don't want matron blacklisting me."

Five minutes later a text arrived on his phone. I only knew this because he had set his phone to make the sound of a ship's horn every time a text arrived. Bugger me it was loud. I don't think he knew how to put it on silent mode.

As his phoned resembled the warning horn on the Titanic, I noticed that the machine connected to the old boy opposite made some very strange noises and the lights on it kept flickering. Then all of a sudden it flat lined and rang out a continuous bleeping noise. All the nurses rushed in expecting to see the old git dead and to administer CPR. Instead he was sitting up reading Train Spotters Weekly.

They all looked puzzled and confused, as did the old boy. The Doctor reset the machine and then checked out the old boys blood pressure, temperature, pulse rate and reflexes. You name a medical procedure and he was having it done to him. He was getting a bit pissed off, because as far as he was concerned there was nothing wrong with him.

"Your bloody phone did that Al," I said.

"No way," he answered, "Impossible."

Ten minutes later and all was calm again. The old boy could relax and get on with reading the article about a train spotter who had sex for the first time, but declared that spotting the Flying Scotsman was far better.

Suddenly Alan's phone went off again. Another text had arrived.

The old boy's machine went haywire again and then flat lined.

This time the chaos was even worse and top Doctors came running in trying to work out what was going on. This time the old boy was pulled, poked and prodded with all kinds of instruments. Not guitars or trumpets, but medical instruments. He was severely pissed off now.

"Fuck me Al, it is your phone doing that," I said.

"I think you might be right," he said, "I'd better turn it off."

"No way pal," I replied. "Leave the bloody thing on. I've never enjoyed myself so much!"

Yes it was cruel, but the old boy was only getting his just desserts. He'd hogged the TV the whole time I'd been here and he was the first to moan about my visitors. What goes around comes around. Revenge is sweet.

I did feel slightly sorry for him in the end though. Alan received five more texts before he left!

Whilst I am writing this chapter, the Medical Association have confirmed that mobile phones do not in any way interfere with medical equipment. Yeah right, well they did seven years ago!

The two days passed and Sarah had come to collect me and take me home.

I thanked all the Doctors and nurses and I said my goodbyes. I gave the middle finger to Dads Army as I left and then I collected my mountainous supply of painkillers from the pharmacy on the way out.

The car journey home was agony. Every bump the car went over caused me pain and what with the state of Britain's roads, there were a hell of a lot more bumps to come. I gritted my teeth and thought about seeing the kids in about thirty minutes. This got me through that painful journey, knowing I would see joy on their faces when I arrived home.

Sarah had told them to be careful when I walked in

through the front door and to cuddle me very gently. However, do kids ever listen to their parents?

I slowly made my way up the drive and opened the front door.

"Dad," they both shouted. They ran over to me, throwing their arms around me tightly.

"We've missed you so much," they both said and hugged me even more tightly.

It bloody hurt like hell, but I didn't show it.

I'd missed my kids so much, but now I was home. Happy days!

Chapter 6
Can Men Have Periods?

The postman dropped the mail through the letterbox. There was the normal crap like bills, credit card statements and a leaflet on how my funeral could be paid for if I started saving now.

Was God trying to tell me something and dropping subtle hints? I'd thought about dying when I was told I had a tumour a few weeks earlier and once whilst I was in hospital just before my operation, but that was sheer panic.

All my thoughts back then were rushed and I wasn't thinking straight.

I was at home now and I had plenty of time on my hands to think rationally about everything.

Leah was at school and Charlie was at playgroup. Of course Sarah was about, she wouldn't leave me all on my own. However, it was springtime and she was busily cleaning every nook and cranny in the house. I had time to think rationally.

Did I have cancer? Has it spread? How long have I got on God's earth? This time I wasn't scared when I asked myself these questions over and over again in my mind. Rational answers kept leaping to mind, however these answers were all maybes and were not for definite.

I would find out the answers to my questions in a few weeks, as one of the letters that dropped on the doormat was confirmation of my appointment to go back and see the specialist in three weeks. Christ, Groundhog Day yet again. I've got to bloody wait once more. Would I re-live the same bloody nightmares that I suffered before?

No I wouldn't. As I said earlier my thoughts and fears were no longer in panic mode. I was very calm and relaxed and thinking rationally. I just prayed that these calm thoughts would last.

Right, if I am going to die, what next. Not for me, but for Sarah and the kids. I know what's next for me. A cremation followed by me shooting off to meet God at the pearly gates. Mum and Dad would be waiting nearby on their clouds, arms outstretched ready for the hug that I have missed for so long. I definitely want to be cremated. Get the job done properly. No way am I opting for a burial. Christ, what if I'm not dead properly. The thought of being buried alive scares the shit out of me. Am I being stupid? Probably, but I bet I am not alone in having these fears.

Right, what would be the next steps for my family should I die? I had to make sure they would be okay.

I hadn't made a will, so that's one thing I needed to do. I'm of the generation who believe you only make your will when you are old and perhaps on death's door.

I'm way too young, there's no way I'm going to die just yet. These were my thoughts before I had my tumour. However, my thoughts were a whole lot different now. I might bloody die.

Making a will is always one of them things you put off and off until it's too late.

Take my work in the bank for example. I've seen too many people affected when their loved ones are gone. Distant relatives then come creeping out of the woodwork to lay claim on the deceased's estate. All because a will wasn't made. I reckon I've seen this scenario over a thousand times during my time at the bank. However, this still hadn't jump-started me in to making one.

It felt like I was saying to God, "Right I've made my will, so I'm ready when you are."

It seemed the longer I put it off the longer I would live.

I know it's utter bullshit, but that's how I felt and I'm sure I'm not alone.

Dad hadn't made a will either and he ended up making his will from his hospital bed just before he died. I suppose that's why I associate wills with being final. I'd seen it first hand with my Dad and it fucking killed me inside. How must he have felt making his will knowing he was going to die? I can't imagine it. I can't comprehend it. It's too painful.

I hate it when people use the words brave and courageous when a footballer steps up to take a penalty. What utter fucking nonsense. Bravery and courage are what my Mum and Dad had, and not forgetting every other person who has fought cancer. Knowing they were going to die, now that's brave and courageous.

However, my wake up call had come. I'm 27 and I might have cancer and die, so bloody get a grip and sort out that sodding will and make sure Sarah and the kids don't go through the pain I suffered when watching Dad making his.

Although Dad did make his will in the end, my brother and I were left with a small mortgage to pay on our family bungalow, as Dad's life cover didn't cover the whole debt. So as well as emotional hardship, there was financial hardship too. Luckily we were both in good jobs.

Fortunately I had plenty of life cover at the time (and still do), so Sarah wouldn't be left with a mortgage to pay. She would also receive a generous pension from the bank. Financially, I had made sure Sarah and the kids wouldn't suffer. They would still have a home they could call their own.

The only thing I couldn't have any control over were

their emotions.

Dad and husband would no longer be around. How would they cope? Who would play soldiers with Charlie? Who would teach Leah to ride her bike? Who would hug Sarah when she felt down? Sarah will move on in life and may well find love and happiness again. She would be hugged again, but not by me. Charlie would play soldiers, but not with me. Leah would ride her bike, but I wouldn't teach her.

These thoughts really hurt me and I started to cry uncontrollably. Then I realised, as tears were streaming down my face, that I was supposed to be rational and getting a grip. Don't take two steps forward and then ten back. I pulled myself together and erased those thoughts from my mind. New images materialised. I was hugging Sarah, I was playing soldiers with Charlie and I was teaching Leah to ride her bike. I need to live and be there for my family in the future. I felt much better.

If I had cancer, then by God I was going to fight it and kick the living shit out of it. I had a job to do, the best job in the world. Being a Dad and a husband.

Cancer may have beaten my Mum and Dad, but I was going nowhere fast.

Well, apart from the solicitors to make my will that is.

I passed my time at home laying on the settee and reading my course work ready for my trip up to Leeds in a couple of days. Although I was still sore at this point, I could see no reason as to why this goal was unachievable. In between reading I took some well-earned breaks and slept.

The stairs at home weren't causing me too many problems, apart from the fact it took me forever to climb the buggers. The hospital had given me some bottles to pee in, just in case I couldn't make it to the bog in time.

I'm so glad they did. Every time I climbed the stairs to go to the toilet, I took a bottle with me in case I couldn't hold it any longer.

There was one occasion where I knew I wouldn't make it. I'd got to the sixth step and I needed to pee there and then. I couldn't hold it a second longer. I suppose drinking a bottle of Lucozade in one go didn't help.

Anyway, down came my pants and trousers. I had the bottle in one hand and my cock in the other. I guided my bell end to the opening of the bottle and I started to pee. Oh the relief. Now I may be alone in this thought, but I think the relief of finally peeing after you have held it for so long is far better than sex.

I suppose I could combine the two, but I don't think my missus is in to all that. Shame, I could get double bubble then.

As I was peeing into the bottle and grunting out huge sighs of relief, the front door opened. In walked the mother-in-law to be greeted by my arse in all its glory. I was also moaning and groaning at how good I felt. What a sight. I was going to turn around and ask her if my tackle looked any different with one bollock, but then I remembered she'd never seen it with two, so she wasn't the best person to ask.

The only person who would know is Sarah (and all the Doctors and nurses in the hospital, but I wasn't going back there). Oh, and of course me. However, I was biased and in my opinion it didn't look any different as I stood naked in front of the mirror. I wanted a second opinion and who better than my lovely wife who's had hands on experience with my tackle at least twice in the last year. Well not quite hands on, just the tips of her fingers! Now you may well be thinking, "Hang on, how could she have touched it twice if you only get it once a year." A fair point I think. Well, once was obviously on my birthday when I got a bit and the second time she didn't know she was touching it. She was doing a sausage casserole one

119

night and she asked me to pass her a Cumberland. For a laugh I presented my tackle instead, which she firmly grasped. However, she had the last laugh as she coolly replied,

"I said the Cumberland not the chipolata." Bitch!

I was going to show Sarah my package tonight in the privacy of our bed. She would then be able to tell me if it looked any different and, more importantly, did it still look like her little Walnut Whip (or has it morphed into an ugly looking mass of foreskin and bollock). I briefed her on her mission and she said,

"I'm only looking at it, I'm not going to touch it."

Yeah okay darling. You haven't seen my nob for a while and I'm confident you'll want a piece of it. You won't be able to resist. You'll be thinking, "Does it feel different? I've got to know."

Besides, I want to know if sex is any different with one. I feel it's only right that my wife partakes in feeling my crown jewels and then asks politely if I wouldn't mind shagging her senseless. Just for research of course. I mean, if it was the other way around and she'd had some work done downstairs, I'd gladly give her one to reassure her that her lady garden was still fit and healthy. It's part of marriage. Part of the vow states, "To have and to hold." Well dear wife, I have this new package and I want you to hold it. She can't back out. It's a legally binding contract and I've got witnesses who heard her say this. I'm onto a winner here. I'm confident that my new look package will lure her in. My nob will be like a Rubik's cube. She won't be able to stop playing with it!

Anyway that was later. I'd finished my pee and pulled up my pants and trousers. I then gave the bottle to Sarah to dispose of. There was no reason now for me to climb the rest of the stairs, as I'd done my business. Besides, by the time I'd have got to the top my pee would probably have solidified and ended up stinking out the whole house. It made sense for Sarah to get rid of it. I tried to make a joke of it so she would at least enjoy this little task.

"See, I told you that you always take the piss out of me," I laughed as she emptied the bottle down the pan whilst holding her nose.

"Christ," she said, "Did you eat loads of Sugar Puffs in hospital."

"No," I replied.

"Well, your pee stinks of Sugar Puffs you big fat honey monster," she shouted sarcastically.

She had a point though. Since then, on several occasions, I have noticed my pee stench resembling a bowlful of sugar puffs. Funny though, because I never eat the things!

The day went and bed time beckoned. I struggled up the stairs, had a pee (still hadn't done a crap since I got home), cleaned my teeth and sprayed my nob with a quick spurt of Right Guard. I felt it only right I present my nob to Sarah in a fairly acceptable state.

I lay down on the bed and waited for Sarah to come in and answer all my questions. Yes, second opinion time had arrived.

She walked in wearing her sexiest nightwear. I knew it. She definitely wanted a piece of my new tackle. Normally she would wear woolly pyjamas and stripy bed socks, but on this occasion she had chosen a little black silky number. My nob immediately stood to attention. My first hard on since my op. Good, it still has feelings, even with one bollock.

Sarah sprayed the bed with some room spray (essence of cucumber and spring onions I think). It definitely smelt like a fresh mixed salad. She sprayed it several times over me. What's she trying to tell me? Perhaps she was going to put two slices of bread either side of my nob and eat it! A sausage salad sandwich. That's definitely not in the Karma Sutra.

This is it. The moment of truth. I performed the sound of a drum roll with my mouth and slowly pulled back the duvet to reveal my package post-op.

"Well?" I said to Sarah.

"It doesn't look any different to me, apart from your pubes," she responded.

That's it; bloody rub it in about my shaven pubes. They had started to grow back, but at that moment they resembled a cowboy's stubble.

"Feel it as well," I said, "You know you want to, you minx."

She reached out her hand (I was hoping for her tongue) and she closed her eyes.

"Bloody hell," I shouted, "It isn't going to bite."

Her hand finally grasped my tackle and she began caressing my lonely bollock.

"Yeah, of course it feels different, there's only one now," she said, "However it doesn't matter. The main thing is it doesn't look any different. It's still my little

Walnut Whip!"

That's what I wanted to hear. I wasn't a freak and Sarah wasn't disgusted or put off by it. Normal service had resumed.

In fact I like to think my package in its post-op state turned Sarah on. Why else would she have dressed up for the occasion? The fact that she actually agreed to touch it was a bloody miracle. She definitely wanted to sample the goods. It may have been sheer curiosity to see if I could still shag with one bollock, or it may just have been her animal urges. Who cares? She wanted a shag! This is it. The moment of truth.

"You'll have to climb on top and do all the work," I said. "I'm still a bit sore to be thrusting back and forth for sixty seconds."

I didn't even finish my sentence and her silky black nightie was off. This one bollock lark definitely has its advantages. She was like a dog on heat.

However, tonight's momentous shag was not to be. As soon as Sarah climbed aboard the bus of love, the pain hit me.

"Aaargh, get off," I yelled.

Now Sarah's not big, in fact she's only a size 10, but that sodding hurt. My wound was throbbing, unlike my nob, and my stubbly pubes were sticking to Sarah's short bush like velcro. It took twenty seconds to prise our love tools apart.

Sex (making love for Sarah's benefit) would have to be put on hold for a while. In the meantime, could my one bollock cope with all that sperm? Well tough shit, he was going to have to. I didn't fancy a wank to relieve myself, as all I kept seeing were my half-shaven pubes. I'm afraid my friend that'll you have to wait till Daddy's pubes have grown back (and you'll have to wait until Daddy's pain free in the groin area as well).

I was gutted and Sarah was gutted. Of course she said don't worry, but I'm sure I heard her mutter, "The sex is still the same then." I apologised to Sarah and then I took some painkillers and drifted off too sleep.

I awoke in the middle of the night, as something didn't feel right down below. I was bloody sore still. I pulled back the duvet and to my horror my boxer shorts and the sheets were covered in blood.

Now I know I am in touch with my feminine side, but I was pretty sure I wasn't starting a period. I wasn't moody or touchy and always shouting at everyone, so I couldn't be on. I was also confident it wasn't Sarah as there would have been no chance of any nookie if she were flying the red flag!

Whilst I'm on the subject of periods, I need to get another thing off my chest. Please bear with me.

It's those bloody adverts on the TV where women are on their period, but because they are using new ultra with wings, they're on top on the world. What horse shit!

My missus uses those bloody things with wings and I can assure you she is in no way on top of the world when it's her period.

Yes, the advert shows a woman gliding down the high street shopping, saying hello to every stranger, smiling at all the kiddies in their prams and generally feeling great. Then she is off to meet her girlfriends (who are also on) for lunch, where they will sit for the next two hours giggling and eyeing up the hunky waiter.

Is this real life? No way! My missus stomps down the high street muttering, "Fuck off," to every stranger she passes. The kiddies in their prams are scared shitless as she pulls the ugliest face she can (not hard to do when she is on). Then she meets her mates ("girlfriend" is so American) for lunch, where they sit moaning about stomach cramps and how heavy their flow is that morning.

That's real life, but of course the sellers of tampons can't show this in their adverts, otherwise they wouldn't sell any.

Where was I. Oh yes, where was the blood coming from if it wasn't my monthly time or Sarah's? The soreness of my wound should have given me a clue. That's where it was coming from. My wound was open and was bleeding. Holy shit I thought. I'm no medical genius, but surely this isn't right. I don't remember the Doctors saying,

"Of course we stitch you up, but in a few days expect your wound to open up and gush out several pints of blood."

I turned to Sarah, who was snoring, and pushed her to wake her up.

"Sarah," I shouted, "Wake up."

She slowly came round, looked at the alarm clock and announced with anger,

"Jesus, it's 2 o'clock in the morning you tosser."

Perhaps she was on after all!

"My wound has opened up and I'm bleeding quite a lot," I replied.

She jumped up with such vigour that her tits whacked her in the face. However, she was now alert and was listening.

I showed her my wound and it was still pumping out

lots of blood. Good job I wasn't living in Transylvania, as this would have been one hell of a buffet for Dracula.

"That's not right, " she said now scared.

"No shit Sherlock," I answered her sarcastically.

"I'll ring the hospital and you er, you just stay there," she said even more scared than before.

Stay there. I was hardly likely to get up and start break dancing!
The hospital had given me the number to the ward I had stayed on in case of any complications after my op.
Five minutes later Sarah came back up the stairs.

"They're going to send a district nurse round in the next hour to have a look," she said now relieved.

"But we don't live in Yorkshire," I replied.

"They have district nurses in Essex as well," Sarah answered.

"Thank fuck for that," I replied.

Okay, so I thought that district nurses only existed in Yorkshire. It's not my fault. I've only ever seen them in Heartbeat and Where The Heart Is. I've seen them driving around the beautiful Yorkshire countryside in old Morris Minor's, immaculately dressed in their uniforms, their hats neatly nestling upon their heads. Somehow I can't picture them driving around the clogged up roads of Essex in a Ford Capri. It doesn't seem right.

Luckily the kids were still asleep, which was good news. I didn't want them seeing all the blood.

We waited downstairs for the nurse to arrive. I had been given a supply of bandages and lint dressing from the hospital, so I used these to place over my wound to stem the bleeding.

Around forty minutes later the district nurse arrived. She was a typical district nurse, hat and all.

It was now around 3 o'clock in the morning. The bleeding had calmed down a bit and it wasn't as bad as when I woke up.

"Right, lets have a look Mr Couchman," the nurse said in a Yorkshire accent!

I showed her my wound.

"Yes, quite nasty," she added. "Your wound is infected."

"Infected," I said with surprise." Where would I have caught an infection then?"

"Could be anywhere," the nurse said, "In the hospital, in the car, or here at home."

I was confident it wouldn't have been at home, as Sarah and I are really hot on cleaning everything with Dettol multi surface cleaner, what with having two young children.

Yes, Dettol multi surface cleaner. It cleans, but also kills 99% of all household bacteria, including e-coli. It retails around £1.39 and is available in all leading stores. What a plug. What blatant advertising. I deserve 10% of all Dettol profits please. If Dettol need me for a new advert, then I'm available.

"I'll clean your wound and then put on a new dressing," the nurse said.

In my confusion, I thought she said she was going to put on a new dress. How odd I thought, but hey she knows what she is talking about. She's probably got blood on her current dress and would need to change in to a new one before she meets her next patient. I became quite embarrassed as I said,

"I'll leave the room so you can put your new dress on in private."

"No," she said slowly and loudly as if I was deaf. "I'll p-u-t o-n a n-e-w d-r-e-s-s-i-n-g."

"Oh sorry, I misheard you," I said apologising.

She carried out the procedure and then gave me a course of antibiotics to clear up the infection and to make it as good as new again.

"You shouldn't need stitches again," she added. "The antibiotics will do the trick."

"Thank you very much," I answered. "And I'm sorry about the whole dress thing."

Mind you, it would've been bloody nice if she had stripped off in my front room. I could've ticked that fantasy off my list entitled, "Daza's top 20 fantasies to achieve before I die." The selfish cow! I might have cancer and die soon. I haven't got a lot of time left to complete the list. The least she could've done was peel off her uniform and move her boobs around a bit. That would have left 19 fantasies to go. However, one of my fantasies may be a trifle tricky. Where will I find a woman with three tits? Bingo, I've just remembered where I can find one. There's one in that Arnold Schwarzenegger film called Total Recall (avid Arnie fans will know what I mean.

If you don't, hire it out and enjoy). Mind you, she is an alien, but beggars can't be choosers when there is a list to complete.

"If you need anything else from me just call," the nurse said.

"Well there is just one thing you could do for me," I replied.

Shit. I can't believe I just said that out loud. I was supposed to think it not say it. My perverted brain had taken over and it wanted me to fulfil fantasy number 20 off the list.

"What would you like me to do?" the nurse asked.

Now control yourself man, deep breaths. Think of something sensible to say back to her.

However, my brain was now making me see her slip off her uniform to reveal black stockings and suspenders. She had a tattoo of the NHS logo just above her belly button. Married to the job I thought. Her dress fell to the floor and she beckoned me over, winking her eye and rolling her tongue around her lips. Oh God, please don't make me say the wrong thing. Big breaths. Yes she did have big breaths! Aaargh. I didn't answer.

"Mr Couchman, what is it you want, I'm a busy lady," she said, now getting really pissed off.

"Erm, er, erm," I stuttered." Would you be offended if I asked you to take off...er..........take off......... er..........?"

"Come on," she said very sternly.

"Take off your hat," I said. "So I can see how wonderful your hair looks."

"Get some sleep Mr Couchman," she replied, tutting and shaking her head as she left the house.

At least I didn't say something stupid!

Now call me a cynic, but I'm pretty adamant I caught this infection from the hospital. As I said before the standard of cleanliness isn't great in lots of hospitals, whereas the standard in my house is way above average.

I suppose I am a bit obsessed with cleaning and I like things neat and tidy also.

This all stems back to when Mum and Dad died. As I said earlier my brother and I had the bungalow to look after. We continued living in the bungalow for a couple more years until it was sold and we both moved on in our different directions.

The bungalow in my eyes was still Mum's and Dad's and everything inside it was still theirs. They had worked bloody hard to make it look nice. I made sure everything was looked after and everything was neat and tidy. No way was I going to let their stuff go to ruin. I constantly cleaned everything to make sure it was all perfect. Day after day, hour after hour. It became such a routine in my life that to this day I still obsess about cleaning.

Sarah moans to me about how I've taken her role of being a housewife away from her, just because I do all the housework. Crikey, any other woman would love their man to put on a pinny and get out the Dyson and a duster. Mind you, I can see it from her point of view. I do undermine her. For example, when she cleans the kitchen worktops I immediately go behind her and I'll do it again, but to my standards. I can see why she gets narked off, but I can't help it. It's in my nature.

I digress again. What was I talking about? Oh yes, my infection. As I write this book today, the well-known infection MRSA is big news. Hospitals say their standard of cleanliness has improved immensely, yet why is MRSA and other deadly bugs so bloody rife? This infectious nasty bastard has actually killed people and to this day it is still killing. In today's paper there is a story about a war hero who died in a British bug-ridden hospital. Not my words, but the newspapers. He survived two wars, three years in a POW camp, was awarded an MBE, yet he died at the hands of a deadly bug that he caught whilst in his local hospital. For his widow and family it's bloody heartbreaking. He only went because he had broken his hip. It's a bloody shambles.

Seven years ago when I was ill, MRSA wasn't as well known as it is today. I'd heard of the term MRSA, but I thought Marks and Spencer had merged with Rumbelows and Asda to form a new company called MRSA. Yes I was young and naïve. The only time I brought a newspaper to catch up on everyday things was when Dear Deirdre's photo casebook in the Sun was hotting up. Why is it that all of these photo casebooks end up with a lesbian clinch, even though it started off with a married couple addressing their lovemaking problems. Look, I'm not complaining, but if they keep spoiling me with lesbo sessions every day, soon I'd become bored with it and I'd switch to the Daily Telegraph instead. I mean, if you eat chicken dippers every day you'll soon become fed up with them and you'll switch to turkey twizzlers instead.

I reckon I'd got this MRSA lark in my wound. Back then I didn't have a clue about this bug and to be fair I don't think the hospitals were aware of it too much either, unlike today.

Thinking back, the district nurse did say it was a nasty infection. Nasty, I reckon the buggar was mental. It had opened my wound up like a tin can and made me bleed heavily. The more and more I think back, the more and more of me reckons it was MRSA. Of course I've got no proof, but I just have a gut feeling and lets be honest, most of my gut feelings have been proved right. However, there is nothing I can do about it now, apart from thank God that it cleared up okay. However, we can't lay all the blame of MRSA at the hospitals door. How many people actually bring nasty bugs into the hospitals by not washing their hands when they enter the wards? Hundreds I reckon. We all need to play our part, not just the cleaners.

The antibiotics the nurse prescribed me did the trick and within a week my wound had healed up nicely. In between there were moments where it did produce the odd bleed now and again, but thankfully the wonders of modern medicine had prevailed over the evil infection.

Now, all the drama of my wound opening up and the district nurse coming out (not out of the closet) happened on Friday night and into the early hours of Saturday morning. The next day I was supposed to be picking up my mate to make the long journey north to Leeds.

All along I was confident of making it, however this sodding infection was a setback. If I'm honest it was only a minor setback. Even if I hadn't caught the infection, I still wouldn't have made it to Leeds. I was still in some pain and discomfort around my groin area and my pubes were itching like mad. There was no way I could drive, it was too uncomfortable, and I was still struggling to walk properly. No, the Doctors were right. I'd had a major op and resting would be the best course of action. To be hundreds of miles away from home on a fairly stressful course would be utter madness. If anything, I'd probably have made things worse. The other obstacle that prevented me from going to Leeds was my appointment in a few weeks to see the specialist for my results. This clashed with being up in Leeds. There was no way I was going to cancel my appointment, it was far too important, and I didn't want to have to wait another three weeks for an alternative one. It would drive me insane.

It was done. I phoned up my mate to let him know the bad news and I then phoned my boss. My boss told me I could have as long as I needed to recuperate. I would then be placed on a new course when I was ready.

Of course I was gutted, but my health took priority over work. I'd be no use to anyone dead, apart from an undertaker, the local crematorium and the obituary column in the local paper.

Looking back with hindsight, it was a good job I decided against going to Leeds. On the Monday I developed a bad cough. It's only a cough I hear you cry. However, I was the one crying. I had a little tickle in my throat and to get rid of it I coughed. All normal so far, except I didn't expect the pain to be the worse I had ever experienced. I shouted out very loudly and Sarah came running in to see what was up. I think she half expected to see me keeled over on the floor and not standing normally as though nothing had happened.

"What's the matter?" she said. "Why did you shout out so loud?"

"I coughed," I replied.

"Yeah okay," she said puzzled. "But why did you shout out so loud?"

"No, you don't understand, it's my cough that's causing me the pain. It's bloody unbearable," I said.

"That's weird," she added. "A little cough can cause all that."

"I know. It's bloody killing me around my wound," I answered grimacing. "Oh no, here comes another one."

I didn't want to cough again. I tried hard to resist it, but nothing could stop my cough from coming. I tensed up my whole body and waited for the pain to hit me.

I coughed and the pain was so harsh. I fell onto the settee crying like a baby.

Sarah rushed into the kitchen to look in the medicine cupboard for some cough mixture. Luckily we had some left over from a cold ridden February.

"Here, take some of this," she said. "I know it won't work straightaway, but over time it should help."

I swallowed it and lay back down on the settee moping.

I had the cough all day Monday and all day Tuesday. Those two days were hell. I'll never forget the pain I suffered with each cough. Knowing what was to come every time I coughed was sheer agony. I must have coughed every two minutes or so. I'm not afraid to admit that I cried a lot over those two days. I can't describe the pain because I don't want to. It's best left alone. I pray I never have to go through that again.

By Wednesday my cough had cleared up and my wound was starting to heal nicely. I was a little sore still, but a vast improvement had been made. The painkillers were still doing their job (although not when I had my cough) and I was getting up the stairs a lot easier with each passing day. It was only when I climbed the stairs on that Wednesday evening to have a slash, that I realised I hadn't had a poo since I'd got home from hospital. Christ, that's around four days now! I'm normally as regular as clockwork. I perform the play "Richard The Third" (that means turd in cockney rhyming slang) without fail every morning at 7.28am sharp.

I suppose so much had been going on since I got home, that I didn't realise my gut was as solid as a rock and that I hadn't been for a poo.

"Why hadn't I been though," I asked myself? "I'm still eating bran flakes every morning. These always do the trick."

After pondering for a couple of hours, I decided to phone the hospital ward for some advice.

"Oh it's your painkillers," said the nurse on the other end of the phone. "Their main side affect is constipation."

Now they tell me. I've been taking the bloody things for four whole days. No one told me this when I left the hospital.

"I recommend you eat lots of fibre and prunes Mr Couchman," the nurse added. "This should start your bowels moving."

Thanks for nothing. I've got a turd the size of a breeze block up my bum and all because I'm taking tablets to help with the pain in my wound. In some ways this counteracts the whole pain killing process. Yes they help with the pain in my groin area, but what about the pain my bum is going to experience when it expands to four times its normal size just to deliver the sodding thing.

Sarah went to the supermarket and stocked up on lots of high fibre crap. All Bran, Ryvita, prunes and wholemeal bread to name but a few. You name a high fibre product and I'm sure I ate it.

The only trouble was I still couldn't go. Five days later and my gut was even bigger. It looked like I had swallowed half of Stonehenge. I was still taking the painkillers, because I was sure that all the fibre I was pumping into me would make me go. How wrong could I be? The only thing the fibre did was to keep making me fart every ten seconds. Boy I wish I could have followed through just once. It was very uncomfortable having not been for a poo for ten days. Oh please Lord let me crap myself.

I decided I would stop taking the painkillers to see if this would help at all. Bingo. The next day I felt ready to go. Operation "Squeeze That Turd Out" was swiftly put into action. I rushed upstairs to the bog and sat down. About an hour or so later, after many pushes and lots of moaning, I had been. The relief was unimaginable, however so was the pain. I reckon I had just experienced what giving birth must be like.

Now I know why Sarah said it stung a bit when she gave birth to Leah and Charlie. Mind you, this constipation lark is no walk in the park I can tell you. I had to sit on one of Leah's rubber rings for the next fortnight!

It would have been handy if that Gillian McKeith from the TV programme "You are What You Eat" were here to analyse my poo. You know who she is don't you? She can tell peoples diets and how healthy they are just by taking a look at their poo.

What would she have made of mine?

"Well Darren, I can see you eat lots of fibre which is good. However I recommend you push your bunch of grapes back up to where they belong and then go and buy some cream for your wee bottom hole?"

Until my appointment was due, I passed my time at home by letting Sarah wait on me hand and foot. I didn't want to see her get bored did I?

I got lots of phone calls from family and friends to see how I was doing. The only trouble was I had to keep saying the same old stuff to everyone, because they were all asking the same questions. I wish I'd taken out an announcement in the local paper explaining how I felt and how I was doing. Then everyone could read it and then they wouldn't need to call me. However, they were only showing that they cared, so it's something I put up with.

I also had lots of visitors each day. Before they came I told them not to bring anymore grapes and Lucozade, but instead bring lots of chocolate and coca cola. If I saw anymore grapes I would have shoved them up their bums, one by one. However, having visitors each day was a Godsend. The days would go so quick. So quick in fact that the day of reckoning had arrived. The three weeks had gone and the day was here. The day that would tell me whether I had cancer or not.

Chapter 7
Is It Cancer?

My appointment was mid-morning, around 10.30am.

My wound had healed up nicely and I was now able to get around okay. In fact I was even able to drive now without any discomfort.

When I got out of bed that morning, I honestly thought I would be shitting myself. However I was very calm, so calm in fact that Sarah became frightened by my odd behaviour.

"Aren't you worried?" she asked.

"No not really," I replied, "I'm ok."

Of course everyone reacts differently. Some people would be really scared, others wouldn't even be able to go to their appointment and some people like me would be very calm.

I think the reason for my calm behaviour was because deep down, in my heart of hearts, I knew I had cancer. Now I didn't know for sure until the specialist gave me my results, but ever since the day he told me I had a tumour, I'd resigned myself to the fact that I had testicular cancer.

Yes I'd cried many times since that awful day. Yes I'd thought about dying and yes there were times I was downright scared shitless, yet it's funny. The day of reckoning had arrived and here I was unable to cry any more tears. I'd used up all my emotions on previous days. Of course, using humour and having a positive outlook had helped me immensely too.

My plan was simple. Stay calm, don't cry, smile and let's just get on with smashing this fucking awful disease to kingdom come. In reality there was a 50% chance I didn't have cancer, but somehow I knew that there wasn't a chance in hell that I would escape its evil clutches. There was just too much stacking up in favour of me having it. My parent's history, a tumour, aches in my groin and bollock and the specialist telling me to prepare for the worst. Christ, he knows what he is talking about. Telling me to prepare for the worst was in fact him saying,

"I'm sorry, but I think you have testicular cancer."

Lets face it. The statistics say that 1 in 3 people will develop cancer at some stage. Well the fucker has already taken two people from my family, so I reckon the sod will want his hat- trick. He'll want the match ball all right and he's looking at taking mine!

The most important factor of all though, was my gut feeling. This had never proved me wrong before.

Lots of family and friends including Sarah would say,

"Don't worry, you've probably not even got cancer."

I would reply, "I'm sure you are right " or "Lets hope so then."

However, I knew they were all wrong, but I didn't tell anyone about my feelings, not even Sarah. They were all so positive; it seemed a crying shame to tell them otherwise.

I was prepared and I was ready for whatever the cancer would throw at me.

Sarah and I arrived at the hospital about 10.15am. That day was beautiful. The sun was shining and the sky was clear. All I could see for miles was blue sky. What a day to be told you have cancer. Mind you, I suppose it was better than having a dark grey sky with rain pissing down and thunder clapping ever so loudly in the distance. That would have topped off a really shit day, having shit weather as well. The sun was shining for a reason and the sky was blue for a reason. To make me smile and to give me a real lift. Thanks God for thinking of me on such a difficult day.

We spent our normal routine of trying to find a parking space, which we eventually found after driving round several times like Nigel Mansell on an F1 circuit. I've never seen so much road rage. One old granny was waiting patiently for someone else to leave their space. The other car drove off and just as the granny was about to edge in, a young bloke in a jazzed up Ford Cortina nicked her space. She was livid! The young bloke just ignored her and went to walk off towards the hospital. However, Granny Smith was having none of it. She whacked him from behind with her handbag and as he fell to the ground she kicked him in the bollocks.

"Now move your heap of a car or I'll rip your bloody head off," she yelled at him as he writhed on the floor in agony.

Up he got and ran back to his car holding his bollocks. He moved his Cortina and quickly drove off. Granny Smith then parked her car and got out.

As she passed me she said,

"Little bastard. I needed that space more than him as I'm here all day."

"You visiting then?" I enquired.

"Oh no, I'm the hospital chaplain and I've got five sermons to do today," she replied.

I was flabbergasted and astounded by the chaplain. I mean, five sermons in one day. That's a lot of sermons.

We passed the lovely duck pond again on our way to the main entrance.

This time a moorhen shouted out, "You probably haven't got cancer."

Bloody hell, has he been speaking to my family and friends?

I nodded back and smiled. He then charged off the grassy bank and into the water without a care in the world. Until a bloody great pike tried to bite his leg off.

We walked into the reception area and I looked up at the board displaying 1001 directions to every part of the hospital.

There were so many ward names, x-ray departments, outpatients departments etc etc, that I didn't have a clue where to go for my appointment. I didn't have a nurse to help me this time.

Just as I was about to give up and go crazy, a porter walked by. I showed him my appointment letter and politely asked him where I needed to go. He pointed to his left and literally the outpatients area was only about twenty yards away. It was right under our bloody noses. He must have thought I was a right nob head.

We walked in to outpatients and I reported in with reception (a rather moody receptionist saw to me, which is good news, as the clinic must be running on time).

She told me to take a seat and that a nurse would call me shortly. Why would she want to call me shortly when my name is Darren? Weird.

Now, you may be thinking that I haven't mentioned the most important thing ever when attending an appointment regarding my crown jewels. Yes, I'm talking about the showering of my package or the lathering up method if time is precious. The biggest rule of appointment attending. Present one's package smelling nice. To be honest, I didn't mention it this time around as I assumed you would all know my ritual by now. I didn't want to harp on about it again. Anyway, for those of you remotely interested, I showered my bollock and nob with Sphinx's new shower gel called Paradise Fruits. It contained essence of mango and grapefruit. Fresh and really fruity.

At 10.30am a nurse called out my name and asked me to follow her. I asked Sarah to wait behind. I know it sounds selfish, but I wanted to do this on my own. I didn't want to see Sarah get upset if the Doctor did confirm my gut feeling. I would explain everything to her afterwards.

I went into the room, shook Doc's hand and sat down. We chatted about how I was feeling and then he checked my wound.

"It's healed beautifully," he announced.

We then got onto the crux of the matter. Have I got cancer or not?

Doc was ready to give me the news...

"Are you sure you don't want your wife to come in and sit with you?" he asked.

"No thanks Doc, I'm okay," I answered.

He looked a bit miffed, but obviously respected my wishes. He then moved a box of tissues nearer to within my reach.

Now that one thing he said and that one thing he did, confirmed to me that I was going to get bad news. Why else would he have asked if I wanted Sarah to sit with me and why did he move the tissues nearer to me?

I suppose most people have someone with them for moral support and then they use the tissues to stem their tears when being told they have cancer. Not me though. I wasn't going to cry. I had made my mind up weeks ago that I had it. I've done my crying thank you; lets just get on with it.

"I'm sorry to say that your tumour was cancerous Mr Couchman," Doc said.

"Ok," I replied, "What's next then."

He was taken aback by my response. No tears and no breaking down. He said it again, "Darren, your tumour was cancerous. You've got testicular cancer I'm afraid. You do understand what I've just said?"

Strange how Doctors use your first name when they need to get some bad news across. I suppose they are trying to be more like a mate than a Doctor and are trying to soften the blow a bit.

"Yes I heard you okay Doc. I've got testicular cancer," I said quite matter of fact. "So what happens now?"

"You've taken the news well Darren," he added surprised.

"I'll be honest Doc. I knew it was going to be cancer from the first day I saw you," I said.

"I don't get many reactions like yours. However, it's good and you seem very well prepared," he stated.

"Too right Doc," I replied. "I'm going to kick the shit out of it starting today. Bring it on."

Doc explained that there are two types of tumour. One is slow growing and the other is a really fast aggressive one. Luckily I had the slow growing one, otherwise I wouldn't have been here today and writing my story. I would've been dead. Doc knew about the local Doctors fobbing me off for eight months or so. He said that if I'd had the more aggressive tumour it would've been goodnight Vienna.

This made me fucking angry. This was my life they'd been pissing about with. I could have died.

He then stated some good news. The cancer was confined to my bollock only and hadn't spread anywhere else. That was a huge relief I can tell you. Thank you God (I'm thanking you so much I feel I need to give something in return. I know, I'll go to Midnight mass every Christmas and become a hypocrite like everyone else).

"Does this mean I won't need any chemo or radiotherapy then?" I asked Doc.

"I'm afraid not Darren," he answered. "Yes, I'm extremely confident you'll make a full recovery, however you will still need some chemo to make sure any remaining cancer cells are destroyed."

Chemotherapy. Shit. I'd seen what chemo did to my Mum. Dad never had any chemo. You'll find out why when you read the final chapter. My biggest worry now was that my wife and kids would see the same things happen to me.

Doc carried on, "The good news with the chemo Darren is that you will only need a one off shot of it."

"So I won't need weeks and weeks of chemo then?" I asked.

"No you won't. Because it hasn't spread and was

confined to your testicle only, a one off shot should do the trick," he replied confidently.

"What about my hair, will I lose it?" I said very nervously.

I've always taken great pride in my hair and sometimes I would spend hours getting it just right. That's my perfectionism again.

I remember one day in particular. I had arrived home from the hairdressers and they had cut too much off. It was way too short for my liking. I couldn't style it the way I wanted. I tried pulling my hair upwards to make it longer, but of course I wasn't a person from the Play-Doh Fuzzy Pumper Barber and Beauty shop (the toy where hair made of play dough magically shoots through holes in little peoples heads to make it look longer). By the way, you can buy this toy on Amazon.com if you want a piece of retro history. Well, it was available the last time I looked.

I was so angry about my hair that I threw my hairbrush into the sink. Trouble was the hairbrush went straight through it, leaving a gaping big hole. My Dad went ape shit and pulled me out of the bathroom by my hair (strangely enough it did feel longer at this point). He kept shouting, "You're going in the army to learn some discipline you bloody idiot."

I learnt a harsh lesson that day. Don't get your hair cut short if you want it long.

Anyway, Doc said, "No you won't lose your hair and you won't suffer any sickness. It's a new type of chemo recently introduced and it doesn't have the nasty side effects you normally associate with it. You may feel a little tired though, but that's all."

"That's a relief then," I said. "At least I won't have to

go through the same shit that my Mum went through."

Of course it also meant Sarah, Leah and Charlie wouldn't see me reduced to someone they wouldn't recognise. I was feeling okay about the chemo when all of a sudden it struck me. I'd read somewhere that chemo can make men infertile. Okay, so we'd got our one of each and the likelihood of us wanting anymore kids was virtually nil, however I didn't want that choice taken away from me completely, just because the chemo had killed off my little tadpoles.

I expressed my concerns to Doc and he advised me to bank some sperm before I had the chemo, just in case. He said he would refer me to a sperm bank hospital in London and that they would contact me with an appointment before my one shot of chemo. That was that sorted.

The next three months of my life were going to be very busy with all sorts of appointments, ranging from banking my tadpoles, having my chemo and checking that any remaining cancer cells had been zapped.

There was no way I could have combined all these appointments with my course up in Leeds. It would've been impossible. Every couple of days another letter would arrive in the post detailing some kind of appointment or another. It was a good job I put my course on hold for a while.

I pretty much knew my timetable now and what to expect over the next three months, however there was one last thing Doc wanted to have a chat with me about before I left. He wanted to talk about my remaining bollock and how I felt with just one.

"We can put a prosthesis into your scrotum," he said.

"What the hell has a Greek Poet got to do with my

bollock?" I enquired.

"No Darren," he answered. "When I say prosthesis, I mean a false testicle. What's your thoughts on this?"

Thoughts? I hadn't even contemplated this scenario. Sarah said my tackle still looked the same with just one and personally I didn't feel any different. I felt quite normal with one. As far as I was concerned it still looked like I had two bollocks every time I looked in the mirror. The only time I notice the true difference is when I'm regularly checking my other bollock for lumps. Granted, medical evidence states that testicular cancer is unlikely to return in the other bollock, however I'm taking no chances. Plus I like fiddling with my knacker and I did promise my remaining testicle that I would look after him extremely well.

"A false one?" I replied, quite taken aback. "What is it then?"

I half expected him to say it was a genuine bollock from a bollock donor, or perhaps a pickled onion would do the job, the only problem being that I would get a raving great hard on every time I saw a cocktail stick with a lump of cheese on it.

"It's made of silicone and is the exact size and weight of a normal testicle," he said. "Some men feel lost with only one testicle and prefer to have a prosthetic one put in."

"I'll need to speak to my wife about this Doc," I said. "Can I get back to you?"

"Of course, give me a ring when you are ready. If you do want it done it's only a small operation and you'll be out the same day," he told me.

Sarah and I had already talked about my remaining bollock in great detail. She was happy, I was happy, so why the need for a false one? Blimey, she even resigned herself to the fact that it would sound different banging against her thighs. Bloody hell, a silicone one could muck it all up. Who knows what sound silicone makes against a woman's thighs? It might sound like a xylophone. Christ, I could end up playing "The Grand Old Duke Of York" whilst in the throes of passion. However, it's only fair I address her on this matter.

"Okay doke Doc. Thanks for all your help," I replied as I shook his hand.

That was it. My appointment was over and thirty minutes had flown by. Doc was so helpful and professional, but more importantly down to earth. I liked this quality in him. I can't stress how good a Doctor he is. I owe my life to him, as do so many others. A top notch Doctor. There was some good news. He told me that I would see him again soon for my next check up. This instilled a huge amount of confidence in me and I knew I was in safe hands. A Doctor I could trust at long last.

I walked over to Sarah and she looked up.

"I've got testicular cancer," I announced.

"Oh God," she replied as tears rolled down her cheeks, "I'm so sorry."

"I'm okay," I said. "Lets get out of here and get a bite to eat and I can explain everything the Doc said."

We made a sharp exit and we passed the same

moorhen on the way back to the car.

He didn't say a word. He noticed Sarah was upset and he just ruffled his feathers and looked away in respect.

How were all my family and friends going to take the news? They weren't as prepared as me. They were all expecting the other answer and for everything to be fine and dandy.

Sarah dried her eyes and she didn't say a word as we got into the car.

Although I was prepared, the appointment had still drained the shit out of me and I needed a pick me up. And what better pick me up than a big breakfast at the local supermarket? They serve breakfast until 11.30am, so I had plenty of time. It's only a five-minute drive from the hospital so that's where we went.

Most people on being told they have cancer would probably want to go home, but not me. Sausage, bacon, egg, beans, tomato and a hash brown were my next port of call.

We arrived at the supermarket and started queuing up in the restaurant. At that time the supermarket was offering a 6, 8, or 10-item breakfast.

Of course I went for the 10-item breakfast. I was really drained and I reckoned my body needed ten items to get it back to full capacity. I had an empty void in my stomach and the ten-item breakfast was selected to do the job.

Whilst waiting to be served I carefully selected ten items in my mind. Right, two sausages, two bits of bacon, two hash browns, beans, two tomatoes and a fried egg. The queue wasn't moving too quickly. Bloody hell! At this rate it will be gone 11.30 by the time I reach the hot food counter and then the spotty student serving will announce with glee, "I'm sorry but breakfast has finished."

Then I'll advise him that I actually arrived at 11.15 and

that if he weren't so bloody slow I would have reached the hot food counter in good time!

Luckily the queue starts moving and I edge ever nearer to the student. It's now 11.25. Come on you twats in front of me. Can't you just have a coffee and move on? Don't you know I've got fucking cancer? Then some fat git in front of me orders a ten-item breakfast and he can't make up his mind whether to have mushrooms or a fried slice. Have the fried slice Billy Bunter and bloody hurry up and pay will you! It's now 11.28 and there is only one person in front of us. Oh no, it's an OAP! We're done for. Might as well start to look at the lunchtime menu, as we've got no chance of breakfast now. However, she only wants a round of toast. Hurrah for the OAP. I take back everything I've ever said about them, except all the stuff in this book.

It's now 11.29 and it's our turn at last. I started to change my ten-items. Shall I have two fried eggs and only one hash brown? Or mushrooms instead of beans? No way I thought, you've got to have beans on your plate. Jesus, what bloody hard decisions I had to make.

I bet Gordon Brown has got it easy in Downing Street regarding his decisions. "Do we pull out of Iraq or don't we?" is not a patch on whether I want brown bread or white?

It was crunch time. What do I want? The student was looking at his watch. Ten seconds till 11.30. After much deliberating I ended up ordering my original decision after all. Now, I'm always careful with these numbered item breakfasts. You've got to count up your items as you go along. Don't trust the student behind the counter to do it for you, because I guarantee he or she will stitch you up and you'll end up with a sausage missing (sounds painful).

I counted up my items till I reached ten and I gave the student a look of, "You can't catch me out mate!"

Sarah ordered a 6-item breakfast. She told me she

didn't feel hungry (but really she can only count to six).

We collected our cutlery and condiments from the cutlery and condiments section (we're hardly likely to collect them from the drinks section are we).

Why oh why are the knives and forks in supermarket restaurants so dirty? I spend ten minutes trying to find a clean set, by which time my breakfast is stone cold. In the end I choose the set that isn't great, but is the best on offer. I then spend the next five minutes vigorously rubbing them with a serviette to try and at least remove some dirt. They're sodding dirty because they are either placed in a clapped out old dishwasher the size of a car, or some uninspired teenager is given the monumental task of cleaning a thousand knives and forks each day. Hardly job satisfaction is it.

We find a table (dirty as well) and sit down. I perform my normal ritual of opening the teeny weeny packets of salt and pepper and then watching as about one tonne of salt granules all land on my sausage at the same time (the sausage on my plate that is).

Those pesky little packets of salt and pepper are like Dr Who's Tardis. They look small, but inside they are enormous and easily hold several tonnes of salt and pepper. I never seem to get time to sprinkle the salt around, delicately covering each of my selected breakfast items with an even amount.

Instead my sausage has disappeared under an avalanche of salt, lost forever.

My next task is to sweeten my coffee. I can feel my blood boiling as I picture myself opening the packet of sugar. These little bastards operate in reverse to their salt and pepper cousins.

I take two sugars in my hot drinks so I select two packets. Simple enough so far? However, do these two packets of sugar impersonate two proper sugars at home? No they bloody don't! I open up the packet and out fall a measly few grains. I do the same with the next packet and even less plops into my coffee. I then taste it. Does it taste like it's got two sugars in it? Of course it doesn't. Two sugars my arse, more like two grains instead.

So then I have to go and estimate how many packets actually equal two proper spoonfuls. Well I reckon about six.

So I get another four packets from the cutlery and condiment section and then I get stares from all the other customers who are thinking,

"Blimey, he's got a sweet tooth, no wonder he's so lardy."

It would be so much easier if I didn't take sugar in my drinks.

Have you ever mistaken the salt and sugar packets because they are both white in colour or because the words salt and sugar are in blooming French (sel and sucre to be precise). Covering a cooked breakfast in sugar (granted not much comes out) and taking two enormous loads of salt in your tea is not a good idea.

Please change the colours and the wording of the packets Mr Supermarket boss. At least make the salt packets luminous yellow and stop buying in bulk from les frogs. I'm sure there is a proper British company out there that can supply you with packets of British salt and British sugar, delivered by British lorries and driven by British men and women on Britain's roads. I'll stop being patriotic now. It's the bloody French again. They keep cropping up don't they?

At least if the packets were written in English I wouldn't make that stupid mistake again. Yes I did french at school, but the only thing I can remember is how to proposition a French tart and tell her boyfriend to piss off. I never studied the joys of Parisian salt making and

Calais's sugar manufacturers.

Don't get me started on the little cups of plastic milk or cream. I think you all know what I am on about. Lets just leave it or I may have a nervous breakdown.

I start eating my breakfast and in between each mouthful I tell Sarah everything the Doctor had said. Just as Sarah dips the end of her sausage into her fried egg, I mention the fact that I want to bank some sperm.

"Nice time to mention that," she says as she puts the dripping sausage down and pushes the plate away from her.

"Not eating it then?" I reply, as I gleefully stock up my plate with Sarah's leftovers.

I suppose my timing could have been better, but hey, I got an extra sausage and an egg out of it!

As I'm eating I deliberately leave a sausage and the two tomatoes till last. Why you may ask? Well read on. I'm telling Sarah about my cancer, the chemo and where I'm going to bank some sperm, yet at this point I didn't mention the false bollock.

She took it all in and I'm glad to say she looked far more relieved than when we left the hospital some thirty minutes earlier. Sarah now knew all the facts and she realised I had a good chance of getting through it.

This is where the sausage and two tomatoes come in to play. I thought that instead of just asking Sarah outright about the false bollock, I'd create an easy to see picture using the afore mentioned items. I believe that sometimes people can make more rational decisions if pictures are used instead of words.

I placed a tomato either side of the sausage to create a nob and two bollocks and I must admit the breakfast nob looked bloody good. Look, I'm not gay, but even I would have munched away on this glorious member.

I wanted the breakfast nob to resemble my package. Granted it wasn't to scale, as the sausage was way too big compared to my dinky toy. The sausage was at least five inches long.

Sarah looked at me puzzled.

"What are you doing?" she asked.

"What do you see?" I said." Open up your mind."

"Well it looks like a nob," she answered.

"Correct for ten points," I added. "But what about the bollocks?"

"Well they're tomatoes," she said quite correctly, but it wasn't the answer I was looking for.

"Bugger me," I replied, "I know they're tomatoes, but how many tomatoes/bollocks do you see?"

"Well one more than you've got," she said sarcastically with a grin.

"At last, praise be to the Lord Jesus," I shouted. "Right, keep that picture in your mind."

I then ate one of the tomatoes.
"Ok, now what do you see?" I asked.

"Well a sausage and a tomato," she replied smiling, "But I know you want me to say it looks like your nob and one bollock."

"Bloody hell you've got it. Eureka," I said clapping my hands.

"Can I just say though that the sausage isn't to scale," she said laughing.

Rub it in why don't you!

"Thank you for pointing that out my dear," I said disappointed, but deep down knowing it's true. I continued, "Right, which do you prefer, the two bollocks or the one bollock?"

"Why are you asking me this?" she said.

"Well Doc says I can have a false bollock put in if I want to," I replied. "I'm okay with just the one, but I wanted to know how you felt?"

"Bloody hell," she answered. "We've already discussed this. Before I even knew you could have a false one I was fine with everything. You having one bollock doesn't change a thing. What's meant to be is meant to be."

"So what are you trying to say then?" I asked.

"That I'm happy with one," she answered.

"Thanks," I said relieved. "I'll let Doc know that I won't be needing a silicone bollock."

"Besides," Sarah added, "You're married, we're happy and it's not as though any other woman is going to get to grips with your tackle and think, Jesus he's only got one ball."

"Yeah I know," I said trying to hide my disappointment. "But you're right. If I was young and single and sowing the seeds of love (a classic Tears For Fears record by the way), then I'd probably want a false one to even the score up a bit and not to feel like a freak."

"That's bullshit!" Sarah said very loudly. "Young or old, if you've only got one ball that's nothing to be ashamed of. You're still a man, not a freak, and in no way does having one ball affect your sexual performance." (Once I had healed up we did manage to have sex at last).

Blimey, where did that come from? She was acting like a counsellor. She's read too many Womans Own.

By now everyone in the restaurant was looking at me and smirking.

Mind you, I didn't care. It was nice to be reassured about the sex thing. I've still got it even with one bollock. I was being silly. Sarah was right. Having one doesn't mean you're going to be less of a performer in bed. It makes no difference at all.

Nothing changes. I'm still a husband. I'm not a freak and no way am I a lesser man.

Hurrah for my one bollock and thumbs down for the false one. I felt like a Roman emperor casting his decision over a fallen gladiator, although in this scenario the false bollock replaced the gladiator.

I felt good and I felt proud as we left the supermarket to make our way home.

Now all that's left is the small task of letting my family and friends know I've got cancer.

Chapter 8
What a Banker

The first people I needed to tell were my sisters and my brother.

I phoned Denise first. She is my eldest sister. I've always regarded Denise as the head of the family since Mum and Dad died; therefore I felt it only right she received my news first.

I've made her the head of the family in my eyes, because firstly she's the oldest, secondly she has lots of grey hair and finally she's lived longer than the rest of us. Therefore she's had more life experience to call on. A fair judgement I think.

When I told Denise my news she was obviously gutted and was very sorry for me. However, she didn't get upset and cry down the phone. Denise is a nurse and has been for donkeys' years. I reckon she used all her years of experience to hold back the tears. Blimey she's had plenty of practice. Nurses must see people dying nearly every day, yet they remain composed and professional whilst carrying out their duties. Of course they shed tears behind the scenes. It's only natural, bearing in mind the work they carry out. Lots of nurses form excellent relationships with their patients and are well gutted if they die. However, no tears are shed in front of the patient's family. I believe Denise went into nurse mode whilst I was breaking the news and this helped her immensely in holding back the tears. Although she is a nurse and knows most things about medical stuff, she knew nothing about testicular cancer (well apart from it affects your testicles, although there is a big clue in the wording!) I think this scared her like it scared me some weeks earlier. We both knew very little about it and it's that feeling of the unknown that scares the living shit out of you.

Of course Denise offered her full support and said, "If there's anything you or Sarah need at anytime, then don't hesitate to ask will you?"

Why does everyone say this over-used line? It's like we are programmed to say it as soon as we hear the words. "I've got some bad news."

No one ever calls on that person's help, but us English are so polite it's in our nature to offer our help to anyone going through a rough patch.

However, Denise did offer her services and I was going to test her out to see if she actually meant help at anytime.

It was 3.30am in the morning and I rang to tell her that I was on the throne and had run out of bog roll. I advised her that I didn't want to wake Sarah up and as she had kindly offered to help at anytime, would she pop down the 24-hour supermarket and stock up on some Charmin for me? Of course it was all lies, but I wanted to see how she would react.

What she said next I couldn't repeat, but suffice to say I now knew her help meant from 9 till 5.

I found out something months later. After I had got off the phone to Denise she cried her eyes out. She genuinely thought I was going to die of testicular cancer.

She told her husband that I was too young to die and that she wished she could swap places with me. This touched me deeply, however there was a big flaw in her plan to have the cancer instead of me. She hasn't got any bollocks, so how on earth she could get testicular cancer is a mystery. However, it's the thought that counts.

I then phoned my other sister Lee. She's very emotional and we weren't on the phone long as she took the news very bad. Lee was round her ex-husbands at the time and she cried and cried on his shoulder until she could cry no more. Again, like Denise, she thought my time was up.

Lee phoned me later that day, after she had calmed down, and offered her full support also. However, she insisted her support would be from 10 o'clock till 5 o'clock (she likes a lay in).

The next person I phoned was my twin brother James, who funnily enough is the youngest of the clan like me. Well, I tell a lie, I'm the youngest really.

James is one minute older than me and boy does he like to remind me. He always says that because he was the first one out, he got the biggest cock. Wanker.

James was okay on the phone. He said his apologies and then asked a shit load of questions on testicular cancer, which I answered as best I could. He too offered his full support, but not on a Sunday, as Sky's Super Sunday football match took priority over any of my needs.

Now I don't know if my brother cried or not. I've never asked. He's a bloke and you don't ask blokes that sort of question.

Yes I asked Denise and Lee, but they're my sisters. And when I last looked they were still women. When I say looked, I actually mean I observed the hair on their heads and the clothes they were wearing, not the other things. Christ, I know I'm a dirty git sometimes, but I'm not incestuous! For a start I don't live in a remote village where no one ever leaves or visits and the only company one shares is with their closest family! (And their animals).

It's strange really. I can discuss emotions with my sisters, but when it comes to bruv I can't do it. I'm scared to know how he reacted and to be honest I don't want to know. Again, it's that bloke thing. As twins we are really close, yet I still can't discuss this subject with him.

Being so close, it would have upset me to know how he felt and if he cried. Of course I'm close to my sisters as well, but being a twin is so different. We've been brought up together, we've done the same things, we've worn the same clothes, we've eaten the same, we've thought the same things and yes we have swapped girlfriends, although one of his tarts realised when she felt my Walnut Whip (the minx didn't have to tell everyone in school though).

We are a mirror image of each other. Everyone tells us so.

Deep down I have a feeling of how he reacted, but that's how I am going to keep it. A feeling and nothing else. If he ever wants to tell me he can, but I'm never going to ask.

The next people I phoned were my aunties and uncles and close friends.

Blimey did British Telecom's profits increase rapidly over the next few hours. I felt physically and mentally drained after telling everyone I had cancer and then answering all their questions.

When I made my first few calls there was genuine emotion in my voice and I was scared at how people would react to my news. However, after an hour or so of saying the same old bloody thing and answering the same bloody questions, I became robotic and switched to autopilot.

My emotions had drained away and I wasn't scared anymore (which was good I suppose). I didn't care about how sorry everyone was. I was drained and I needed a break. There's only so many times you can say, "I've got cancer," before it takes its toll on your mind and body.

I asked my aunties and uncles if they would pass the news on to other members of my family, save me making any more calls and becoming even more drained.

I also asked the same of my close friends and work

colleagues. The grape vine in this instance would be a help and not a hindrance. Boy does the grape vine work fast! It was the day after I had told everyone and I popped into town just for something to do. I bumped into one of my regular customers from the bank.

We were both in the chemists at the time, shopping down the womens hygiene section. Sarah had asked me to get some of them bloody tampon things with wings that I talked about earlier on in my story.

"They're in a purple box and it must say regular flow on it. Oh, and they must say string panties on the box as well," she explained to me before I left.

"Are you sure they are easy to find? God help me if I bring the wrong one's back," I replied.

"You'll be fine," she answered, "Even a monkey could find the right ones." Great. That filled me with confidence.

So there I was, surveying every kind of tampax, tampon, lilets, towels and pads. Stone me, how many different types do you women want for Christ's sake? Surely you could all use the same thing. I mean, all you do is shove it in your knickers, let it absorb your monthly outgoing of claret and then throw it away down the bog, subsequently blocking it. How hard can it be? But no, they have to be different shapes and sizes and do different tasks. There are ones for light flow, regular flow, medium flow, heavy flow and gushing raging waterfall flow.

Then there are the special ones for when wearing thongs and the standard ones for when wearing big Bridget Jones knickers. Jesus, no wonder you women are moody and touchy when you are on. It must drive you insane trying to choose the right one.

If us men ever had periods it would be so different. We'd just shove a load of bog paper in our pants.

We'd also be bloody proud of our heavy flow instead of just moaning about it, feeling sorry for ourselves.

I can see it now. England are in a penalty shoot out against our old foes the Germans. The world cup is at stake. A well-known England player steps up to take his penalty. Bang! Top corner and we've won the world cup. The player is interviewed after the game.

"You look on top of the world. Tell us what was going through your mind when you stepped up to take the crucial penalty," asks a reporter.

"Well I knew which way I was going to hit it, but you'll never guess what happened just before I struck the ball?" he would reply.

"What?" says the reporter in anticipation.

"My bloody period started," he would answer.

"Blimey and you felt okay?" the reporter asks.

"Never felt better. In fact I would like to say how proud I am to have won the world cup for England whilst having a period," he adds.

And bingo. For the next five years he'd be the face of tampons on the TV and on all the billboards across the country.

I mean, how many women have won anything whilst on? Well we don't know because they've never said. However, us blokes would shout it from the rooftops.

Now ladies, before you find out where I live and cut my last bollock off, I would like to point out that I'm joking. I'm glad us men don't have periods, mainly because it would mean we could get pregnant. I don't fancy that giving birth lark. Nine months of having a large gut and making excuses that I can't do anything because I ache is not for me. Although Sarah would argue that I'm pregnant all the time!

Anyway, I pick up what I think are the right tampons and as I drop them into my basket the customer from the bank said,

"Hello Darren, nice to see you up and about."

"Hello Mrs Smith," I replied. "How are you keeping?"

"Don't worry about me dear, I'm fine," she answers. "More importantly, how are you doing after your operation?"

Blimey I thought. She's only a regular every Wednesday morning and here she is in the chemist's knowing I've only got one bollock. However, things would get worse.

"I'm okay thanks Mrs Smith. I've got time off work to recover and soon I'll be having some chemo," I said.

"It's a shame dear. A young man like you fighting cancer and having both your testicles removed," she replied.

What did she say? Did I hear her right? Both testicles removed?

"I haven't had both removed Mrs Smith, just the one," I stated.

"Oh, are you sure Darren?" she said quite matter of fact. "Only Julie from Somerfields said you'd had both removed?"

"I'm quite sure," I replied.

It was at this moment that I realised, although the grape vine was good in spreading the gospel according to one bollock, the grape vine also worked like Chinese whispers.

Over a period of a week people either assumed I'd had no bollocks removed, or I'd had one bollock and half my nob removed. Someone even thought I'd had the lot removed and was now a transsexual! I bet Leah spread this rumour. They also assumed that I had bowel cancer, prostrate cancer and testicular cancer all in one go. The worst assumption of all was when people phoned Sarah to offer their condolences on my passing. One of my mates fainted when I picked up the phone and answered it!

I need to place another ad in the local, but this time to tell everyone I was alive and kicking. Next time I'll just have to persevere and tell everyone myself, rather than rely on the grapevine.

The days passed and my appointment had arrived for me to go to London and bank some sperm. I felt like Dick Whittington, although I wasn't going to see the Queen. I'm sure she wouldn't have appreciated me masturbating in front of her. I would have been sent to the Tower.

My Uncle Joe, a stalwart eastender from Canning Town, was going to come with me. Let me re-phrase that. Uncle Joe was going to accompany me. I would be the only one coming thank you very much.

Yes, he was along for the ride to support me, but having a wank himself would be taking the support thing a bit too far. Uncle Joe also knew London inside out and he knew the best way to get to the hospital. He's 73 years of age and he's lived in London all his life, so I trusted his knowledge of the London transport network.

We arrived at the hospital just in time for my appointment. We'd got lost on the London Underground and we also went to the wrong hospital. So much for 73 years of experience! His excuse was that he'd never visited central London much and stuck mainly to East London instead. Now he tells me!

The hospital that we went to by mistake was a college hospital for medical students to learn their profession. The one I actually wanted was around the corner, however they all look the bloody same to me.

The problem was I didn't know it was a college hospital for students when I first walked in. Uncle Joe waited outside whilst I went in. I reckon he knew it was the wrong hospital and sent me in so he could have a bloody good giggle. It was a bloody suicide mission.

I only realised my error after I had made a joke with the receptionist.

"Good morning, I'm Mr Couchman and I'm booked in for a wank at 11 o'clock sharp," I said smiling.

At this point I assumed the receptionist had heard this many times and would instantly know that I was actually here to bank some sperm.

"I beg your pardon?" she said very sternly.

"You know luv, I'm here to spank the monkey," I replied laughing.

"Is this some kind of joke?" she added.

I now tried to be serious and replied, "Okay, okay. I'm here to bank some sperm." I then shoved my appointment letter under her nose.

"You'll have some trouble doing that here Mr Couchman," she said. "This is a hospital college for medical students."

Bugger. I wanted the ground to swallow me up. To top it all, there was a load of young student girls queuing up behind me laughing their tits off.

The receptionist continued, "You need to go around the corner. You can't miss it."

"I'm very sorry for the misunderstanding," I said. "Please accept my apologies?"

"It's fine," she answered. "You're not the first one to come here thinking this is the right place. Well not actually come here. They come around the corner in the correct hospital."

She was now pissing herself laughing. The cow. She was playing with me all along (not literally speaking I must add) and I fell for it hook, line and sinker. God she must enjoy her job, toying with poor blokes minds. Mind you, if I were in her position I'd do the same.

I walked out very sheepishly.

"Blimey, that was quick!" Uncle Joe said grinning, but trying to look surprised.

"It was the wrong bloody hospital," I replied. "That's a college hospital and the one I want is actually around the sodding corner."

I knew he was pissing about with me, but I didn't let on. I didn't want to give him the satisfaction of knowing that he had won.

"So you haven't done it yet?" he asked.

"Of course I bloody haven't," I snapped at him. "I'm

hardly likely to produce my sperm in a room full of students am I?"

"Come on," I continued, "Lets just get to the right place."

We walked around the corner and were confronted by another building that sort of looked like a hospital. Was it the right one though? I didn't want to walk in and find out it was a children's hospital of all places. Seeing a grown man tugging at his todger would definitely put the kids recovery back a few weeks.

Outside the main door, either side of it, were two large pillars. Rather oddly, they were phallic shaped. Is this the right hospital? What more of a clue did I need. This must be it. The two great erections standing proudly outside does give it away a bit.

In we walked and I went straight to the reception desk. I just said good morning and handed the receptionist my appointment letter. No way was I going to be making any more jokes today.

"Take the lift to the fifth floor," she said, "And report to a nurse when you arrive."

We got into the lift and up we went. On arrival at the fifth floor I found a nurse and she told me to take a seat and the Doctor would be with me shortly. Uncle Joe went off to find the canteen and get a cup of tea. Whilst I was waiting, I wondered what the procedure for banking sperm would actually be like. I've always had an idea in my mind what it's like and bearing in mind this is the NHS, it wasn't a pretty picture.

I'd probably have to lock myself in a tiny room, pick up a porno mag to get me hard and in around twenty seconds my sperm would be swimming in a little plastic container. I'd then clean my nob with the tissues provided and then toss them on top of the pile of used tissues that are overflowing from the bin in the corner of the room. This was my vision of banking sperm under the NHS.

Uncle Joe came back with some tea. I couldn't drink mine. I was too nervous. What if I couldn't get it up? This wasn't my normal comfort zone to get an erection. I had no problems getting it hard in the bedroom or in front of the computer, but this was an alien place to me. Would my pecker be too shy to come out and play? I could be in the room for hours. Then there's the added pressure of whether I can produce enough tadpoles to fill the container, or would I under perform and just dribble a few drops instead. I don't want to hand the container back to the Doctor with hardly anything in it. I've got my macho image to uphold, even with one bollock. If I didn't produce enough then I'd have to do it twice.

"Hello Mr Couchman," the Doctor said, "We are ready for you now."

"Okay Doctor," I replied. "You wait here Joe."

"Well I'm not coming in there with you!" said Uncle Joe.

I say some bloody stupid things when I'm nervous.

"Right Mr Couchman, first I need you to fill in some forms for me," Doc stated.

The forms were all about why I was banking some sperm, how long I wanted it kept frozen for and if I died did I want them destroyed. Of course I wanted them destroyed if I popped my clogs! They are a part of me. I want to be like a Viking and make sure all of my personal belongings die with me. I did have the option of letting Sarah use them should I die, but it just didn't feel right to me. The thought of my kid being raised without his or her Dad, whilst I sit on a cloud in heaven playing with Gods knockers, is bad enough. But having never held or kissed him or her, well that would kill me inside.

I've already written about my fears of not seeing Leah and Charlie achieve certain things. There was no way I was going to let another kiddie be added to the equation.

I signed the forms and now I was ready. Doc handed me a small plastic container and guided me to a room.

"Okay Mr Couchman. Once in the room lock the door behind you. Then you can get on with producing a sample into the container," he said. "There are some pornographic magazines on the table if you need them."

Christ, that's one part of my vision that had come true. Lesbian porno mages to help me along. Nice touch from the people of the NHS.

As I entered the room, Doc said one last thing. "If you need any help at all please go and see nurse Jackson* in the room opposite." * (The name has been changed to protect that persons identity). I've always wanted to say this!

Any help? What does he mean by this? Will she help me get hard? Is she going to do it for me? Now, if I were going private this would be standard practice I'm sure, but this is the NHS. Surely to God I wasn't going to get a free hand job from a nurse in uniform.

I eagerly looked in the room opposite to see what nurse Jackson looked like. Nurse Jackson was a big fat bald man, first name Ronald. Thanks for the offer Doc, but I'm pretty confident I can do this job for myself.

I locked the door behind me. The room was fairly small and all the walls were white. I suppose they were this colour to cover up any splashes and blobs caused by a sudden volcanic eruption from some blokes pecker.

I walked towards the table in the middle of the room. There must have been around twenty porno mags laid out on the table, all open at different pages, but all displaying the one thing guaranteed to get me hard. Naked women. My earlier thoughts of, "Will I get it up?" vanished immediately. I didn't rush in and grab the first mag on top of the pile though. No, I wanted to choose the right mag and also the right woman. It's not everyday I get to masturbate over a porno mag whilst banking some sperm. This moment had to be special. I wanted to savour the ambience of the occasion. I flicked through a few mags trying to find my perfect wank partner. There was even a porno mag with men in it. I suppose the NHS need to cater for both sides of the market; otherwise they'll be done for discrimination.

However, I must point out that this mag was not for me, even though I admitted earlier that I would eat a nob and bollocks made from a sausage and two tomatoes.

A few minutes later I found her, or should I say them. Lindsey and Michelle naked on the centre spread of Jugs weekly.

Lets just say that they looked like really close mates and were extremely polite to each other. Oh, and they liked their fruit and veg as well. They definitely eat their five a day, but not through their mouths. Does this count still?

Down came my trousers and pants and up stood my Walnut Whip. I warmed up Mrs Palm and her five lovely daughters. Bloody hell, I didn't want to get cramp just as I was nearing the finale.

I commenced. Sixty seconds later my container was half full. This was fine by me and saved me having to do another one, although I could've easily carried on all day. You should have seen what Lindsey did with twenty cherry tomatoes. Mind you, you should've seen what Michelle did with forty spring onions and a parsnip!

Anyway, the girls did the trick. Thanks me darlings. Our time together was nice, but hey, don't call me, I'm married.

I screwed the lid on the container and grabbed some tissues to clean up. Now where is the bin? I don't believe it. Another part of my NHS vision had come true. There, in the corner, was the bin overflowing with used tissues. An untidy great mountain of tissue and spunk had been formed. I chucked my tissues on top of Mount Cum. No way was I going to push loads of used tissues down into the bin, just so I could get mine in.

I knew exactly where they've been and what's on them.

So there I was. I'm standing in a small room with white washed walls and my whole vision had come true. Lesbian porno mags and an overflowing bin. You couldn't make it up.

I pity the poor cleaner though. Mind you, at least at the Christmas party she can say she's never short of spunk in her life.

I pulled up my pants and trousers and made my way to the door. I would've liked to cuddle the girls and had a fag after our incredible session, however there were three reasons why I couldn't.

1. You can't cuddle a mag (believe me I did try).
2. I don't smoke, never have and never will.
3. I had to give my sperm sample to Nurse Jackson pretty quick so that he could shove it in the freezer before my tadpoles perished.

So there was no time for all that post-sex crap. I waved goodbye to the girls and went out through the door.

I handed my container to Nurse Jackson and off he sped to bung it in the freezer, where to this day it still sits frozen solid.

Uncle Joe looked up and said, "That was over pretty quick. I thought it would've taken longer?"

"What do you mean?" I asked, taking offence to his remark. "Sixty seconds is a bloody good time."

"Well you know," he said.

"No, I don't know," I replied.

"Injecting a needle into your bollock and then syringing out some sperm," he added quite serious.

"You are joking?" I said.

Sadly, he wasn't joking. He was deadly serious. I suppose it's his age.
"Bloody hell Joe," I said. "They don't syringe it out, I had to wank into a container!"

"You what?" he shouted. "You mean I've got up really early, travelled all the way to central London and got lost in central London, just so you can have a bloody wank?"

"That's about the size of it," I replied.

He just shook his head in disbelief. We're from different generations and in his day I suppose masturbating was looked upon with disgust.

To this day, as I write this book, I've never had to use my frozen tadpoles and I never will. Why you may ask? Well Sarah is pregnant and we're going to have a little girl. In fact it's due any day now as I write. Buggar, two weddings to pay for now. Now I know I said earlier that I didn't want to add another kiddie to my family, however this one wasn't planned, but as you know with me, things happen for a reason. Perhaps it was God's way of saying I wasn't infertile and that the chemo hadn't affected me. Well whatever, I think this gives hope to any other man who has to go through the shit I've been through. Of course you still need to bank some just in case (and get to meet Lindsey and Michelle for starters), but I'm living proof that there's a chance you won't become infertile and you can hopefully go on and produce wonderful healthy children.

I know it's an expensive way to find out I'm not infertile, but hey, at least I can say I made a kid with one bollock. Not many men can say that and boy do I tell everyone and shout it from the rooftops. And when my little girl is old enough, I'm going to make damn sure she knows she was made from just one bollock and indeed how special this makes her. Of course Leah and Charlie are also very special, however they originated from two testicles.

This little miracle is something I would never have dreamed of happening after what I'd been through. However, hope springs eternal and with this comes hope for every man who has to undergo chemotherapy and worry whether they can make a baby or not. As the saying goes, "Keep your pecker up." I did and look what happened.

When I told Uncle Joe about Sarah being pregnant he said,

"Bloody waste of time going to London all them years ago."

Cheers Unc.

Whilst I'm on the subject of my missus being up the duff, I want to put the record straight on something. Sarah has said that I have taken no interest in this pregnancy whatsoever. She has brought loads of magazines about pregnancy and she is gutted that I've not even read one word. Utter crap. Only the other day I read an informative article on the best sexual positions for a pregnant lady. Very interesting. I've also taken a great interest in her now firm boobs and enjoy popping into Mothercare to peruse through mountains of silky bras. I've also asked her how long it will be before we can have proper sex again. With my fat gut and her ever-increasing tummy, well it's bloody impossible to do the missionary position. I just keep rolling off! "What about all the other positions you've just read about," I hear you cry. Leave it out will you. We're married. They don't call me Mr Missionary for nothing. Oh, and I've also asked her at what point does the milk stop coming out of her breasts. There are two reasons for this.

1- Once the milk stops, then comes the bottle-feeding. This will mean I have to take my turn. Bugger.

2- I'm fed up getting a mouthful of sour milk every time I indulge in some foreplay with her jugs (this only happens right at the end of the pregnancy. So don't worry new Dads. You can still suck away in the early days and not have to worry).

And I was there at the conception. What more does she bloody want? Women eh. You can't live with them and you can't live without them. Anyway, enough about my pregnant wife.

When I got home that night, tired and weary, Sarah told me that the hospital had rung and my chemo appointment was on the 5th of June.

Great. One day before Charlie's birthday. There was no way I was going to cancel the appointment, as it was way too important. This is my life we are talking about.

I couldn't take the chance of re-arranging the chemo session and having lots of little cancer cells zooming about my body for another month or so. However, I was really worried about how I would be feeling for Charlie's birthday party.

I was fine for Leah's a few weeks earlier, as I'd healed up nicely and was able to do things normally again.

The trouble was that my mind was painting pictures again. What if I was too tired or sick to enjoy his birthday? I started to feel guilty and I hadn't even had the chemo yet. Yes the Doctor had said it was a new chemo drug and I wouldn't suffer any sickness, however I wasn't convinced. I could only associate chemo with sickness, tiredness and loss of hair, purely because I had seen it first hand with my Mum. I tried to tell myself otherwise, but it's fucking hard when all those awful memories kept flooding back into my mind.

There was only one way to find out if the chemo was going to affect me and that was to have it and get it over with.

I went to the hospital with Sarah and my eldest sister Denise. As I mentioned earlier Denise is a nurse and I wanted her with me because of her medical background. If any jargon came up during my conversation with the Doctors and nurses, Denise would be well equipped to answer any of my concerns. Not that I anticipated any jargon cropping up, because all the Doctors and nurses I had met previous were very professional and explained things very well. However, I wanted Denise there just in case. In a way she was also taking the place of Mum who, had she still been here, would have insisted on coming with me, fussing and wrapping me up in cotton wool.

Okay, the real reason Denise came was because she wanted to do some shopping in town after my session.

My chemo appointment was roughly six to seven weeks after my initial operation. I would like to congratulate the NHS on the way they had dealt with

175

me. From seeing the specialist to having the chemo, all the Doctors and nurses were excellent. However, the biggest thing I would like to applaud them on was the speed at which things moved. Everything happened so quickly. I'd heard so many negative things about NHS waiting lists and I thought things would take months and drag on, yet seven days after seeing the specialist I was in theatre having my op. Now that's what you call a good service. I've waited longer queuing up for the Next sale on a cold December morning.

Mind you, having a lump that two Doctors missed probably helped speed things up a bit.

However, my good fortune shouldn't distract from the fact that there are still long waiting lists in other areas of the NHS structure, yet the Government doesn't seem to give a shit. MP's harp on about what changes they will make and how better off the health service will be, but it's all bullshit. Nothing ever changes and nothing is done.

Only yesterday I read in my local newspaper about a pensioner (yes he also fought in the war) having to wait two years for a hearing aid on the NHS. He's put his life on the line for freedom, yet he has to wait a totally inappropriate length of time for some help. If he were an illegal immigrant he'd probably get one straightaway. And have a new house and car thrown in for good measure.

So much for freedom, this poor bugger is a prisoner in a world of near silence.

We've got thousands of homeless people sleeping rough in the UK, yet we give houses and flats to immigrants who arrive at our shores pleading political asylum. Now don't get me wrong, I'm all for helping the genuine immigrants who have fled war torn countries, however the trouble is we let in too many people who just want a better life and know that this country will give them free hand outs. Jesus it makes my blood boil.

This country is going down the pan and more and

more people are emigrating to better places. It upsets me because I'm a patriot. Although times are bad, I wouldn't contemplate leaving the green rolling hills of Clacton on Sea. I'm proud to call myself English but for how much longer?

We all arrived at the chemotherapy unit and a nurse directed me into the ward.

Oh how my heart sank when I walked in.

I saw men, women and teenagers sitting on their beds, receiving their dose of chemo, all hoping that this drug would help them beat the shit out of their cancer.

Some looked really ill. One lady was extremely thin, her face pale and gaunt and wretched with pain. Her hair had fallen out also, the result of many chemo sessions.

However, she smiled at us all, said good morning and wished me all the best. This brought a lump to my throat. Christ, she clearly had so many things to worry about, yet she made the effort to greet me and wish me luck. What courage, what strength. It was like looking at Mum all over again. No wonder so many cancer sufferers beat this horrible disease or at least have a few extra years in life. It's their courage and their will to fight. For some people this is the best drug to have. Sure chemo helps, but I believe that fighting it head on, having the belief to win and laughing in the face of cancer can beat it in the end. I looked around the room and everyone had this in abundance. Stay positive, look on the bright side and make sure you don't start going down the road of negativity. Otherwise the cancer has won.

Many of my fellow patients looked ill and really frail, yet when they smiled it was like their cancer had left their bodies, just for that brief moment. There was hope in their smiles, not just for themselves, but also for every other person fighting cancer and for their loved ones who pray every night hoping for a miracle.

I've felt really proud on many occasions in my life,

yet this one ranks as one of my highest. All this made me more determined to stay positive and above all smile and even laugh. I'd laughed before in the face of cancer some weeks previous with my mate up in Leeds, so there was no reason why I couldn't do it again. Bring it on you piece of shit and I'll give you a right pasting.

I sat down on a chair next to my bed. First, I had to have yet another blood test and this would be sent away for tests. They can tell an awful lot from your blood, the most important for me being whether any of those sodding cancer cells had remained behind. Also I'd have another test about a week or so before my first proper check up to see if the chemo had done its job properly.

Fingers crossed the chemo will work and make sure the cancerous cells all leave home for good.

The nurse took my blood and now I was ready for my dose of chemo. She fitted a candular to the vein on the top of my left hand and then connected a tube to it. This tube led upwards to a drip that contained the chemotherapy drug. It's basically a clear liquid that is slowly fed around your body, hopefully killing any cancerous cells in its path.

I was only having a one off dose, however I would still have to sit there for around two hours whilst the drug slowly left the drip and entered my blood supply.

I asked the nurse if she could set up another drip on my other hand, but instead of drugs, could she pump neat vodka around my body to make me feel more relaxed. However this wasn't possible, as she only had gin. I hate gin.

Eventually, after a couple of hours, the drip was empty and I was full. It was pretty boring just sitting and waiting. However, this was me finished. Mind you, some of these poor buggers had to endure this every week for months on end.

Yet they still smiled as I left and again they all wished

me luck. If you want to meet a genuine hero then go and visit a chemo ward. I defy you not to feel touched and genuinely moved. A truly inspiring place.

Denise wasn't needed to explain any jargon, as the nurses were so helpful. Good job really as she buggered off into town whilst I sat around for those two hours having my chemo!

A nurse gave me the direct phone number to the ward and said that if I had any problems with the chemo, then I just needed to call them or pop in at anytime.

I really felt like I was being looked after and this made me feel good about myself and gave me a huge lift.

The only down side of the chemo was I didn't get to show the nurses my nob and bollock. Apparently they didn't need to see it. I'd shown every nurse in Essex my package over the last few weeks, so why should the chemo nurses be any different? I did offer to show them, but they politely declined.

Shame really. I'd gone to a lot of trouble freshening the little bleeder up that day. I used another new brand by Sphinx called "Volcanic Eruption." Mind you, it burnt my nob red raw. Another brand that won't catch on.

I felt fine as I made my way home. I didn't feel sick and I didn't feel tired. However, it had only been thirty minutes since the drip had finished, so I suppose I was being a tad optimistic. Any side effects would probably take hold over the next few days. It was a waiting game to see if I would suffer from any of them.

The next day was Charlie's birthday and in the morning I was fine. I watched him open his presents and it was a joy to behold the smile that enveloped his face every time he unwrapped a gift. I was so glad just to be here, alive and well, doing the normal things that Dads do on their son's birthday.

Later on that afternoon it was Charlie's party. Nothing big, just a huge marquee, about a thousand of his close friends and an enormous buffet prepared by Jamie Oliver. Oh, and I'd managed to hire Busted for the music and disco. Bloody hell, I must stop trying to be an A-list celebrity. Okay, so the party was under a gazebo, the only guests were close family, the food was from the corner shop and the music was Now 50 blaring out of a crappy tape recorder.

By now I was feeling tired and I had lost my appetite. The appetite thing didn't bother me as the mother-in-law had prepared the buffet and I didn't fancy getting salmonella as well.

I kept dozing off in the armchair. The tiredness had taken over. I tried to shrug it off, but my body wouldn't let me do it. I felt like shit, physically and emotionally. I couldn't join in the party games and I couldn't share in the happy atmosphere of my boy's birthday. I just managed to stay awake to sing Happy Birthday and to see him blow out his candles on his Thomas the Tank Engine cake. Then I went back to sleep. I was so tired. Luckily I didn't feel sick, that was until the mother-in-law brought round a tray of vol au vonts with crab paste sticking out the top. However, I had experienced something that Mum went through. The tiredness was unbelievable. My whole body just gave up and cried out for sleep and there was not a sodding thing I could do to prevent it.

I even turned down my favourite dessert. Now that just isn't me.

However, there was some good news the next day. I felt fine again and I felt normal. I was as fit as a hamster on a spinning wheel. Only one day of tiredness and so far my hair was still intact. Boy was I the lucky one.

I felt so bloody good that I wanted all my future hospital appointments now. The way I was feeling, I would've breezed through them without a care in the world.

Trouble was, the most important appointment of all

was in three months time. The appointment that would tell me if I had kicked the shit out of this fucking cancer.

What was I going to do with myself for three months? I wasn't at work, so how would I pass the time?

Then I thought back to that day when I was told I had a tumour and possibly testicular cancer. The day I didn't know which way to turn to for help.

An idea popped into my head.

"I'm going to raise awareness of this bloody cancer and make sure no other man has to suffer like I did," I said to myself out loud.

That was my mind made up. Blimey was I going to be busy.

Chapter 9
Magazine Superstar

I was really pissed off when I couldn't find anything out about testicular cancer. Who could I ask to find out more about it? Why are there no leaflets in the hospitals or Doctors surgeries? Why oh why is this terrible disease that affects so many men each year not high profile? (Bear in mind that I'm talking about seven years ago. Of course it's very different today).

These same questions kept going over and over again in my mind. I was determined to make sure that no other man would have to go through the same agony that I did. That horrible feeling of being all alone and confused.

I had time on my hands for a few months, so why not make the most of it?

I was going to raise awareness of testicular cancer in a big way. That was my goal and by Christ did I put my heart and soul into my new project.

I sat down at the table and started to think. How could I raise awareness? What shall I do? Who do I get involved to help me?

Then I thought of something. The idea that came to me was ambitious, but hey, what the hell. Lets go for it.

I started to jot down a few notes and then I brainstormed my idea. Around an hour later my idea was ready and all I had to do now was draft it up properly.

I'll try as best as I can to describe my idea to you. Basically I had designed a poster. The poster had four famous sportsmen on the front of it, all lined up in a row.

First there was a footballer, then a rugby player, followed by a cricketer and lastly a tennis player. All of them were holding the type of ball that is used in their particular sport. However, here comes the crafty bit. Their relevant ball was held in one hand and placed directly over their tackle. In the other hand they would be holding a magnifying glass and they were using this to look at their ball more closely.

Above their heads, in big bold writing, would be the caption,
"Lads, don't forget to inspect your balls regularly."

Now at this time no one else had thought of this idea. I'd never seen it done before. I asked family and friends and they also agreed it was a first. With the profile on testicular cancer being so low, this was no surprise. There were no campaigns, no posters, no leaflets, no magazine or newspaper articles and lastly no TV coverage.

I wanted high profile sportsmen on my poster as I felt this would appeal to most men and of course get the message across. Oh, and the fact that they used balls in their chosen profession did help somewhat with the slogan.

I suppose I could have just gone with ordinary blokes dressed up, but I didn't think this would gain enough attention and publicity. If I wanted to raise awareness in a big way then I needed to think big. I'm sure more people would take notice of a poster if it had a famous England footballer on the front, rather than some bloke donning a football strip and a wig.

How would I, a humble banker, get such big names involved in my project? This was a huge task and something in which I would need a helping hand.

So I sent drafts of my posters, along with an accompanying letter explaining my project, to several large cancer charities, the biggest being Cancer Research UK.

This was my plan. The charities would like my idea and they would use their influence in attracting some famous sportsmen to take part. My longer term plan was that testicular cancer would then become much more high profile because of the poster. In turn, this would help men learn more about this illness and, in doing so, not feel so bloody helpless.

I had impressed myself. The whole thing from thinking up the project to sending off my posters took one day. Yes one day. I'd given myself a few months to sort out my project, yet I needed just twenty-four hours. I think it was pure determination and having a will to succeed that spurred me on. Thinking back to that fateful day when I was all alone and re-living my emotions time and time again also played a big part.

All I could do now was wait and see what responses I would get back.

Because I had successfully finished my project in one day, this still meant I had two months and thirty days to go until my first proper check-up appointment. To pass the time and combat my boredom each day, I would potter about in the garden. Nothing too strenuous, because if I overdid it I would get sharp pains in and around my scar area.

The weather was fantastic that summer and it began as early as June. In fact it was so nice I just sometimes lay in the garden soaking up the rays. After a week or so I was really tanned and resembled someone who'd just come back from Spain. It wasn't till my brother James said,

"Bloody hell bruv, you're in the middle of fighting testicular cancer and now you want some skin cancer as well?"

I then realised what I was doing to myself. I was so wrapped up in a getting a nice colour to make me feel good, that I completely and blatantly ignored the risks involved.

You know how it is though. Other people always say how well you look when you're tanned and to be honest I wanted people to say this to me, especially after my last few hellish months. I wanted to feel good about myself and at the time this felt right.

However, James was right. The last thing I needed right now was another type of cancer to battle.

I took his words on board and started to act sensible. I was still outside in the sun; however this time I used a high factor sun cream for protection and I also limited my time in it. Thankfully I didn't have to apply any sun cream to my head, as my hair was still intact and hadn't fallen out. What a relief.

I'd been bloody stupid, like so many others in this country. Skin cancer and the dangers of the suns rays (and sun bed rays too) are big news every summer and so they should be. Campaigns are everywhere. TV adverts spell out the dangers every day and there are plenty of daytime TV programmes that cover this topic too.

So why do thousands of men and women continue to put themselves at risk like I did? Because of peer pressure that's why. If you're a milky white colour in the hot summer months, then everyone says how ill you look. We've all got to be bronzed Gods or Goddesses. We see our favourite celebs and all the top models looking wonderfully tanned and we all want to look like them. Men and women will put themselves at risk because our society dictates that we must look the brownest of all. It boosts our egos. We can show off more skin and wear more revealing clothes. When I've picked the kids up from school in the summer, the playground is a mass of tanned mums all wearing the skimpiest shorts they can find. It's like a competition. Who can be the brownest and wear the skimpiest tightest shorts in existence. Don't get me wrong, I'm not complaining, far from it. A throng of sweating MILF certainly hits the spot for me (if you don't know what MILF means then watch American Pie or search it on Google). However, I wonder how many of these mums use sun cream for protection and stop to think of the dangers? Not many I reckon. It's a strange world we live in. We all want a nice tan for a couple of months, but at what price. I admit people look good with tans, but try telling that to the thousands of people who thought they looked good until they died of skin cancer. A few months in the sun or under a sun bed can seriously harm your health.

We all say it won't happen to me, but so did the poor buggers who are now six feet under.

I'm going to be much more sensible in the sun from now, otherwise I might just become another statistic.

A week or so had passed and still I had no replies from the cancer charities. I admit I was getting a bit stressed about the lack of envelopes falling on my doormat carrying good news.

Two weeks then passed and some letters fell through the letterbox. I could see the names of the charities on the postmark. I eagerly opened them, full of hope, but at the same time extremely nervous. My heart sank when I read their replies. To cut a long story short, they thanked me for my idea and for the time I had put into it, however at this moment they wouldn't be able to help me get my poster up and running.

What's wrong with these people? Surely they of all people should know testicular cancer needs to gain some high profile coverage? They could do something about it, yet here they were unwilling to get involved. I felt betrayed and I felt despair.

I'd been kicked in the teeth and it hurt like hell.

I admit I moped around the rest of the day feeling

sorry for myself, but more sorry for all the men that would be affected by testicular cancer in the future.

There was a small glimmer of hope though. I still hadn't heard back from the biggest cancer charity, Cancer Research UK. Perhaps they would be willing to work with me. No news is good news as they say.

However, the next day there was still no letter from them. I started to wonder if it had even reached them or whether it was at the bottom of a pile of letters in someone's office.

I was ready to sue the Post Office for non-delivery when the phone rang. It was a lady from Cancer Research. She introduced herself and told me she was in charge of the media department. They'd got my letter and were very impressed with my desire to raise awareness. She said my poster idea was great, but at the moment they didn't want to pursue this any further. Instead, would I like to become a media volunteer for them and get my message across in this way? This would involve me doing articles on testicular cancer through magazines, newspaper, radio and TV. It would work like this:

For example, a magazine would approach Cancer Research and state that they want to do a piece on testicular cancer. Cancer Research would then contact me to see if I was happy to do the article. If so, they then put the magazine in touch with me and we would take it from there.

I was well gutted that my poster wasn't going to become a reality, however at least I could still raise awareness by becoming a media volunteer. In the end it didn't matter how I did it, as long as I had the opportunity to get my message across. Cancer Research gave me this chance and I took it. They scratched my back and I scratched theirs.

The lady also agreed that testicular cancer had very little coverage compared to other types of cancer. She stated that Cancer Research were going to do their utmost in making sure testicular cancer would be placed high on many peoples agenda. As long as they had media volunteers like me, then their job would be so much easier.

Mind you, I wouldn't get a gig straightaway. She stressed how patient I would have to be. The charity wasn't allowed to approach the various media channels asking them to do a piece. We had to wait for them. Bloody hell I thought. Testicular cancer is not talked about enough already, so why on earth would some mag or newspaper show interest now?

There was nothing I could do. I would have to wait. I'd spent the last few months doing just that. Waiting for this and waiting for that. Christ did it piss me off and now I would have to wait all over again.

For Gods sake! I wanted to talk about my experience now, not two years down the road!

I even contemplated doing the poster on my own, but after hours of deliberating I admitted defeat and agreed that this was way too big a project for me. Nowadays the use of famous sportsmen and their chosen balls are widely used in raising awareness of testicular cancer, so someone must have taken notice of my poster.

A month or so passed and suddenly there was a turning point in my quest to spread the gospel according to one nut.

A couple of well-known footballers had got testicular cancer and of course this made the news. Obviously I was gutted for them, because I knew what they were going through. However, on the account of them being famous, testicular cancer had made the news and all of a sudden it was being talked about. Testicular cancer was now big news and in every pub and club in Britain, men were now starting to talk about their bollocks.

It's a funny old world. If these footballers hadn't got testicular cancer, then we would've been back where we started. No coverage and no one talking about it. However, they did have it and it got the ball rolling (no pun intended).

Bingo, this was what I had been waiting for.

A week or so later Cancer Research phoned me and asked if I would like to do an article for a well know men's health magazine. Do bears shit in the woods? Of course I wanted to do it! I'd been waiting ages for my chance to tell my story. No way was I turning down this opportunity.

The lady reporter from the magazine phoned me later that day. She wanted to come down to Clacton-on-Sea that Sunday with her photographer.

She suggested that if the weather was nice we could do the piece on Clacton seafront and get some nice photos for the article.

Blimey. That means people walking by will see me getting photographed and will probably stop and stare, wondering what the hell I'm doing.

"Who the heck is he?" they'll all say.

"I'm the man with one bollock. Wanna feel?" I'd shout back.

Carry on walking you nosy gits and let me get on with my photo shoot.

Crikey, I sound like a Z-list celebrity. Now I didn't become a media volunteer to get recognised, I did it to tell my story. However, this still didn't stop me from getting up really early on that Sunday to try on every item of my wardrobe. I also spent hours trying to get my hair just perfect. I used every one of Sarah's moisturisers to make my skin look fresh and supple. If I'm going in front of the cameras then I want to look the part. Anyone else would do the same, wouldn't they?

The time had come and the reporter and photographer arrived. The weather had suddenly changed from being gorgeous to bloody terrible. There was a strong north wind blowing and it was freezing. Now that's what you call a typical English summer. Clacton seafront was a no go. The photo shoot would now be done in my back garden.

Now in all honesty I expected them to be here for about one hour max. Record my story on a Dictaphone, take a couple of snaps and be home in time for Songs of Praise. Simple.

It was only when the photographer started lugging loads of equipment from his van that I began to think otherwise.

He took about thirty minutes to get everything out and then another thirty minutes to rig up it all up. The biggest thing he rigged up was a light. And boy what a light it was. It was a bloody monster! Like the floodlights you get in a football stadium. Now I know today was gloomy and overcast, but this light when switched on would bring a Boeing 747 in to land.

Whilst he was busily setting up, I told my story to the reporter. All done and dusted in twenty minutes. Excellent I thought. Ten minutes of matey snapping away and I'll be inside in the warm before you know it. However, the photo shoot beggared belief. I'm no David Bailey, but even I can take twenty photos in about two minutes. However, the two minutes turned into two hours. Two hours to take some fricking photos and I'm not even famous!

They wanted Sarah and the kids in on the photos, but Sarah hasn't got a photogenic face and Charlie was playing up and being a little sod. This left Leah to join me for the photo shoot. Bloody kids. The article is supposed to be about my bollock, yet there's going to be thousands of readers saying, "Isn't she just the cutest?"

Yes she may be cute, but so is my bollock!

The photographer wanted Leah and I to have the photo done against our garage wall, which basically ran into our back garden. The long garage wall had a door in the middle and a single window towards the right. The window was done out in horrible white nets. This was only done because a room had been partitioned off inside the garage and made into the kids playroom. The nets were to give the kids a sense of it being a proper little playhouse. You may be thinking why on earth I am describing the garage to you in great detail? Well, this becomes clear later on.

Now of course the door and the window would make it into the photo also. Nothing strange about this you may ask. Just wait though and read on.

We took our places either side of the door ready for the photo. Was the photographer ready? Course he bloody wasn't. He wasn't happy. The photo looked bland. He then asked if I would put a few plant pots alongside the wall to brighten things up. Of course pal, I'll do all the sodding work whilst you make sure you don't get cramp in your trigger finger.

Right we were ready and we were freezing. Freezing my bollock off I was (always wanted to say that since my op). Leah was shivering too.

Then he switched on the monster light. I could see the lights dim in our house and the power to the TV drained away. The worse thing of all was that he'd plugged the bloody thing into our mains. I bet the electricity company were pissing themselves laughing as the knobs on my meter went round really quick.

Mind you, the light did serve one good purpose. It gave out so much heat that we instantly warmed up.

Two hours later and my electric bill was higher than Blackpool's illuminations. We were still standing against the wall waiting patiently, but instead of being cold we were now sweating buckets.

We had to stand this way and we had to lean that way.

Smile, then don't smile. Fold your arms, then unfold your arms. Change my top and change my trousers. Move the plant pots and then put them back again. I know people like to take great pride in their profession, but this was taking the piss!

I thought about being a prima donna and charging off set shouting, "Now look here luvey, I didn't have this crap with Woman's Own!"

However, as this was my first gig I thought better of it.

He kept snapping away, then saying he wasn't happy, until at last he said,

"Right this is it. Perfect! The snap that will paint, in the minds of our readers, the story of Darren's fight against testicular cancer."

How the hell would a picture do this? Did he want me to hold a placard above my head saying, "I've got testicular cancer." Or perhaps drop my trousers and pants around my ankles whilst I held my meat and one veg proudly in my hands. They would later add a speech bubble coming from Leah's mouth saying, "My Dad's only got one testicle."

No, please don't do the photo this way!

It's bad enough all the Doctors and nurses in Essex having seen my nob, but not thousands of readers of a well-known health mag as well.

Although on the plus side the makers of Walnut Whips would probably sign me up to do several TV commercials. Sales would rocket.

What he actually meant was that I put a reassuring arm around Leah, give out a great big smile and this would say to the readers, "Yes I'm happy and I'm alive."

"A perfect picture of a loving Dad cuddling his little

angel," said the photographer.

Yeah right. We're talking about my five-year-old daughter, who's going on sixteen and with a vocabulary that's associated with a moody teenager.

The photographer pressed the button on his camera for the last time that day. He was done. The photo shoot had finished. We said our goodbyes and off they went. I was knackered, but at least my story would be told.

I couldn't wait for them to send me a preview copy of the magazine before it hit the shelves.

A week later it arrived. A caption on the front read, "Inspiring stories of men and their fight against cancer."

I quickly flicked through the pages until I found Leah and I standing in full glory against our garage wall, smiling like the cats that got the cream.

The story was just how I told it (I'd heard sometimes they add bits on which aren't true, just for excitement).

I was so proud of the article as were Sarah and the kids.

As I scanned the page I suddenly realised they hadn't put my name under the photo. The other six stories all contained names, but not mine. Marvellous. Two hours of being moved around like a puppet and they forget my name!

However, as Sarah rightly pointed out, who cares. I've told my story and I was raising awareness of testicular cancer. My original goal had now come to fruition. Mind you, the name thing still bothered me. I later told all my family and friends that I wished to remain anonymous to avoid unnecessary fame and fortune!

One thing bothered Sarah as well. The photo. It actually looked like we'd had our photo taken in front of a really small run down house, with off white nets in the window and paint peeling off the front door. The pretty plant pots didn't help either as this made it look like the front of a house. It looked like my shit hole of a garage was in fact my home!

I actually live in a nice three-bed semi in a village. However, the photo gave the impression I lived in a shantytown in Peru.

Bugger.

There's no way now I was going to get any groupies outside my home in Little Clacton. They'd all think I live in South America and go off to Peru. Some old Peruvian git would take all the credit and he'd be signing their breasts instead of me. Tosser.

Come on Darren, calm yourself. Get a grip. Remember it's awareness you seek not fame, although the whole tit-signing thing would have been fab!

Mind you, I think it only best if I practice signing some boobs, just in case a group of birds do happen to come my way. Now, where can I find some large tits? Of course, the answer is right under my nose so to speak. I'll sign my own man boobs for practice (or "moobs" as they are affectionately known in the man boob community).

Once my first piece of media work had been and gone, the phone didn't stop ringing. It was Cancer Research again and again. I was really chuffed. I was getting many opportunities to tell my story and in many different ways as well. Between Cancer Research, the many media volunteers and myself, we were firmly putting testicular cancer on the map.

Over the next six months or so I did articles for the local newspapers, one for the national paper the Daily Star, a piece for a woman's mag called Family Circle and I appeared on Cancer Research's sponsor form for a big charity cycle ride that year.

I was as pleased as punch with all of them. Each one was different in its own way, yet they all shared one thing in common. Raising awareness.

Mind you, the Daily Star did worry me at first. They

said my article would appear in their centre spread. I was worried I'd have to appear naked (as the centre spread rules dictate) and lay down on a Persian rug whilst delicately stroking my one remaining bollock. Generations of my family would be well offended. However, it turned out their weekly health spot always appeared in the centre pages of the newspaper. I would still be on my aunties and uncles Christmas card lists after all.

It's a bloody good job I didn't have to appear naked. I'd been busily practising signing my moobs and the sodding ink was permanent. I suppose I could've have said it was a tattoo. Only trouble is how many tattoos have you seen saying,

"Thanks for a wonderful evening my moob friends. Love Daza xx."

I would have been lynched and placed in the stocks for loving my own tits!

If I was really proud of my efforts then you should have seen my family and friends reactions. They were all dead chuffed. I just hope Mum and Dad would've been proud. Everyone told me they would be. As much as I appreciated my family and friends kind words, I wanted the public's reaction to be the best of all.

Had I achieved my original goal along with the excellent support of Cancer Research? Well, I'm going to go out on a limb and say, "Yes I bloody did." Testicular cancer was now high on everyone's agenda.

I had people coming up to me in the street saying,

"Aren't you the bloke in the Daily Star with only one bollock?"

"Yes that's me," I would reply with great pride.

I've had numerous women friends approach me

about their sons finding something down below. Is it a lump? Aren't they too young? What should they do next? These were questions I was only too pleased to answer and hopefully put some worried minds at rest.

I know I'm not a Doctor, but having experience of testicular cancer doesn't half go a long way when you are talking to other people about their fears. People actually come to see me first before they go to their Doctor. I feel like bloody Jesus, but unfortunately I don't have the healing hands. Although there was one time when I was a teenager. I started going to church because I fancied a girl who went regularly. As the weeks went on I became more accustomed about what to do and what to say around the church going community. For example, I couldn't say, "I don't sodding believe it! This Jesus bloke was strung up for a few days and he still came back from the dead," or "So Mary wasn't shagged by Joseph then?"

I was eventually accepted after repenting all my sins (this took five Sundays in a row).

Whilst out with my mates one evening I pulled a girl who had one tit bigger than the other. A lot bigger. I know because I saw them bouncing oddly as she balanced on my balls one night. Yes I know all about the sex before marriage thing within the church, but let's face it; I only went to church so I could goose some bird in the pews. I wasn't going to follow all the rules, and besides, it was a bit late on the no sex front. I'd already lost my virginity way before I could turn water into wine and all that crap.

Anyway, I told her about my church duties and that I could help her get them to the same size with the help of my healing hands. Bloody gullible she was. Every night for one hour I massaged her smaller tit with my hands whilst saying the prayer,

"Please Lord make this girls tit increase in size."

Something did increase in size every night, only it wasn't her tit!

After about four weeks she saw through me and told me to sod off. Shame. I feel I was getting somewhere in helping her, as I'd found the name of a good plastic surgeon in the area.

Anyway, enough of my healing hands, otherwise the union of GP's will have me crucified for nicking their patients.

Suffice to say, the public reaction was good and I felt I had played a part in this.

Each year more campaigns were launched by the big charities and each year more and more famous people became involved, all wanting to help in some way.

I remember one year the men's clothes store Burtons selling t-shirts to raise money for a testicular cancer campaign. One t-shirt carried the slogan, "Bollocks to cancer." Each year the big cancer charity called Everyman does a massive campaign to raise awareness. They attract some bloody big names as well. Like Cancer Research, they do a fantastic job.

TV programmes like Emmerdale and Christmas Lights have had storylines about a main character having testicular cancer. Last year the actor Martin Clunes appeared in a one off drama about a man's true story of his fight against testicular cancer. Bloody good it was.

Lance Armstrong, the famous Tour de France winner, has suffered from testicular cancer and he's raised awareness of this big time.

Quite rightly, testicular cancer has been placed at the top of the list, along with the other main types of cancer. Hopefully blokes know more about it now and hopefully they're not scared to go to the Doctors anymore. Hopefully they know how to feel for a lump and how often they should inspect their bollocks.

Even if one bloke's life is saved because he had the

courage to go to the Doctor's after reading my story, then I'll be happy. One life saved is better than none at all.

There is one media piece that I haven't mentioned yet. I've left it till last as I feel it's the best piece of work I've been involved with during my media volunteer years. Also I feel the reader always remembers the last bit of a chapter better than the middle bit or first bit. Of course I'd like you to take in every word I've written, otherwise I've wasted my bloody time, but in case you haven't then please take this next bit in.

I did a piece for DIPEX, an Oxford based charity backed by many other well-known charities. Cancer Research put me in touch with them and I thought it would just be another magazine article. However, this was so different to all my other pieces of media work.

The aim of DIPEX was to launch a website covering lots of different types of illnesses, including testicular cancer. The website would contain all sorts of information on the illness concerned, but more importantly it would contain real life stories of people who wanted to share their experiences. Like me for example. I would talk about how I found my lump and what symptoms to look out for. I would discuss any tests I had done and how the specialist came to diagnose my illness. Then I would cover my operation, the chemo and any side effects of the treatments. I would also talk about my thoughts regarding the choice of having a false testicle and the impact the cancer had on family, friends and myself. The last topic I would cover would be sex and fertility.

So basically DIPEX were going to put my story on the Internet and not in print as I had first thought. Normally I'd say not to use the Internet if you are looking for information on a type of illness. There are far too many sites that will just scare monger you. You'll come off the computer twice as worried as before and probably think you've got another three or four illnesses to boot. It can scare the hell out of you. I only know this because I used this method when I knew nothing about my cancer. I logged on to some poxy site from America and ended up thinking I had another type of cancer because of the symptoms I was displaying. I later found out that some idiot, who had no knowledge of cancer, had made up this site. Yet here he was, allowed to set up a website with no backing whatsoever and scare the shit out of worried human beings. It's not bloody right.

However, sites from registered charities like DIPEX are an excellent tool. They use individuals like me to tell my story and hopefully in return answer any questions or concerns.

DIPEX wanted the website to work like this:

They would use a video camera to film me telling my story. This is then placed on the website and the idea is you can click on my link to see and hear my story being told. If you prefer not to see my ugly mug talking to you then you can just click on the text and read that instead. If you don't want to read the whole text then you can just click on certain questions and hear or read my answer. The site would also contain factual information on testicular cancer, its available treatments and links to support groups, organizations and other sources of quality information. Brilliant idea. Choice for the consumer. It sounded bloody good and I was very keen to get involved. The Internet was becoming more and more popular, so it made sense to raise awareness in this way.

Yes I'd done mags and newspapers, which were a fantastic experience, but they get thrown away after a few days. The Internet doesn't. It's there for a very long time.

Different people from all over the world can look at the website and hopefully get something from it. A global audience. Some little bloke in India could get to know all about me. Although most of the blokes that live in India know all about me anyway, as they tend to ring me every bloody night. This was definitely the way forward in raising awareness to a new level. There was no way I was going to miss out.

I did my piece and waited in anticipation for the website to be launched.

Seven years on and I'm still on the website, albeit looking a lot younger and slimmer.

Now when people ask me questions about their bollocks I can direct them to the DIPEX website, www. dipex.org. I can then pop up on their computer screen discussing how I found my lump and what happened next.

Fingers crossed, DIPEX will continue for many years and add more illnesses to its website. Take a look for yourself and you'll be amazed at what a fantastic effort DIPEX have put into this site.

Long live DIPEX and may it continue to help thousands of people year after year.

I haven't done a media piece for a long time now. Blokes with more recent cases of testicular cancer are telling their stories now. It's better like this, as nowadays there are more advanced treatments to speak of and many different procedures compared to when I was ill. It doesn't bother me that I'm old news now. As long as there are blokes out there willing to share their experiences to keep testicular cancer in the news, then I'll be happy.

I had been so busy telling my story that I didn't realise it was only a week to go until my appointment for my first proper check up. The weeks had flown by.

This would tell me if my cancer had gone for good and that hopefully the chemo and my will to live had shone through.

I hadn't even given this a passing thought, as I'd been

so busy being photographed and interviewed.

However, my media work had now finished. I had time to think again.

Have I kicked the shit out of it, or do I need to reschedule another fight?

Chapter 10
Alive and Kicking or Dead and Buried?

Now I was counting down the hours to my first real check up. Every minute of every day my mind was filled with images of how my life might be after my appointment had been and gone.

Don't get me wrong, I was still full of positive vibes, but sometimes I just couldn't stop my mind from wandering over to the dark side every now and again.

Everyone who knew me must have thought how well I was doing in dealing with my testicular cancer. I was smiling all the time and I was using my sense of humour in abundance. However, on the inside, no one could see how I felt. I felt confused and I wasn't sure what the future held for me. Night times were the worst. I kept dreaming two different dreams. One dream was uplifting, whilst the other was a nightmare. I tried to get rid of my nightmares by thinking about Lindsey, Michelle and their vegetable games, but it was no use. As much as I visualised seeing aubergines swallowed whole, my nightmare always appeared when I went to sleep. You can't control your dreams can you? They just happen. I didn't mind the uplifting dream though, as this was full of happy scenes. It's just a shame I couldn't dream this one every night.

My uplifting dream would always be the same. I walk out of my appointment, having received good news about my cancer and feel so alive. I'm bursting with energy and I jump up and down, punching the air with my fist and shouting, "Yes I'm alive!" at the top of my voice. People stare, but I don't give a shit. The weight of the cancer has been thrown from my shoulders and I can start living again. I arrive home and hug Sarah and the kids. Tears of joy and relief flow from our eyes. I phone up all my family and friends and tell them the good news. Who cares about the sodding phone bill? I'll gladly pay it because I'm alive (also it's a dream, so it doesn't matter how much the bill is because I'll never have to pay it). My dream then continues. I'm going out with the kids on a bike ride to the park. I push them on the swings as high as I can. The laughter and the joy on their faces give me so much satisfaction. I'm so glad to be here and so glad to do such simple things that brighten up my whole day. My future looked bright and full of hope. Something my other dream didn't possess.

This was my nightmare. My cancer has spread and the diagnosis isn't good. I only have a few months left and the Doctor's told me to try and enjoy the remaining time that I have.

My dream then switches to me at home. I'm alone and I'm planning my funeral. What coffin do I want? Should people wear black or not? What songs shall I have played whilst the curtains close around me forever? Gone. No more Darren. Dead for all eternity.

The dream then suddenly changes and I am looking down from up above. Family and friends file out of the crematorium, heads bowed and their eyes stinging from their tears. I can see Sarah and the kids being hugged by just about everyone present.

Aerosmith's "I don't want to miss a thing" plays quietly in the background. I'm helpless. I can't do anything and I can't say anything. This is my funeral and all I can do is watch from the spirit world. My dream continues. Sarah is lying on our bed crying. I lie down beside her and put my arms out to embrace her. She can't feel me though and she remains all alone. I'm next to her, but only in spirit. I long to touch her properly and to talk to her, but I can't. I want to stem her tears, but it's impossible. I'm angry and upset. Why did this happen? What have I done wrong? Why couldn't some murderer or rapist die instead of me? Tears run down my face and I scream out...

I always woke up at this point in the nightmare. I think my body couldn't take anymore emotional crap and told my brain enough is enough.

I tell you what though. This fucking nightmare scared the shit out of me. What if dreams come true? Granted, the uplifting dream could come true, so I had a 50/50 chance. As much I was being positive, I couldn't help but let the nightmare affect me.

I even went as far as looking through our CD collection to choose some other songs that could be played at my funeral. I made a list of all the stuff Sarah would need to do when I'm gone. Stuff like how to pay the bills, how to work the lawnmower and how to put water and oil in the car.

These were just a few things. Simple things really that I took for granted, but things that would be difficult for Sarah to do when I'm gone. Simple things that are a chore when I'm alive yet become a longing when I'm dead.

If my nightmare were to become true, at least I would see Mum and Dad again, albeit a little sooner than I had planned. I wasn't actually scared of dying because I knew Mum and Dad would look after me. However, I was scared for Sarah and the kids. Difficult and emotional times lay ahead for them all should I snuff it. Bloody hell, I can't die just yet. Imagine all the grief I'd leave behind. Christ, it would be a catastrophe.

It was these thoughts and a vision of Mum and Dad

that made me pull myself together.

As I was making out the list for Sarah, I sensed someone was in the room with me. I looked up and saw Mum and Dad as clear as day. I was bloody shocked I can tell you. Christ, I'd moved house twice since they died, so how the fricking hell did they know where I lived.

It was so good to see them and I wanted so much to reach out and hold their hands. However, I didn't get a chance to reach out. They spoke a few words and then they were gone. The words they spoke were, "You're not coming with us yet Son. Stay positive and have no regrets."

They were right. I always listened to Mum and Dad and just because they were no longer here didn't mean this would have to stop. If they wanted to get their message across via the power of the spirit world then I'd bloody listen and take notice.

I screwed up my list and chucked it in the bin. A surge of positive vibes suddenly surged through my body and gave me a tingling sensation all down my back. Fuck the nightmare and all hail the uplifting dream.

I looked through our CD collection again, but this time to play an inspiring song for now and not for my funeral. I put on Queen's "Don't stop me now" and I played air guitar whilst singing into a banana. I felt good. Thanks Mum and Dad for looking out for me. Lets put our meeting on hold and I'll see you many years later.

Every hour that I counted down to my appointment was now full of positive energy and thoughts.

I didn't have the nightmare anymore. The only dream I had now was the uplifting one (and occasionally Lindsey and Michelle appeared carrying a punnet full of strawberries). It was so nice to wake up each morning and have a smile on my face and look forward to the day ahead.

Bring on the appointment because I'm bloody ready

for it!

A week or so before my appointment I had the customary blood test. As I said earlier, this one was to check that the chemo had worked and killed off any remaining cancer cells.

I chose to have this done at the local blood clinic instead of making an appointment and seeing the nurse at my Doctor's surgery. You didn't need an appointment at the clinic. You just turned up, collected a number from the receptionist and waited for your number to be called.

The clinic opened at nine in the morning, so I decided to get there at around quarter to, thus avoiding any long queues. When I arrived I was gob smacked. I'd never seen anything like it before. There was a queue a mile long, all full of old age pensioners. They were all chatting to each other about the good old days when you could leave your back door open, let your kids out to play all day long and collect your pension with a pension book.

I've seen pensioners queue before, like outside the post office and outside the newsagents when the new edition of Seventy Plus comes out. However, this was something else. A hum dinger of a queue. I reckon I had a good hour wait before I would be seen.

Why do all the retired people have to get up really early and be first in the queues? Bloody hell, they've got all day long to get their bloods done. Okay, so you are now shouting out that I had got all day long too, seeing as I was off work. It's a valid point, however I would be going back to work very soon and then it would be different. I'll only have an hour's lunch break to get my bloods done in the future, yet their lunch hour is at least ten hours long!

Christmas time really gets my goat. It's the last day before the supermarket shuts for Christmas Day and Boxing Day. Just a mere two days to every sane person, but to an old duffer this transforms into two weeks. As far as any old age pensioner is concerned, the shops will remain closed until the middle of January. However, the rest of us know they will be open again the day after Boxing Day.

Guess who are at the front of the queue a good thirty minutes before the supermarket doors open. Yes you've guessed it, Cyril and Maud. It gets worse, because in Maud's hand is a list a mile long, which means they are going to stock up on two weeks worth of groceries. Every old duffer in existence buys up every last item on the shelves within the first hour of the shops opening. This means that every other human being that visits the shop after their shift is finished is buggered. There's nothing left, not even a breadcrumb. All because the old duffers brigade have to get in the queue first. It's nearly eight o'clock in the morning and Cyril is wielding the trolley like it's a weapon. He's ready to barge anyone who dare get in his way when the manager puts his key in the door. However, this is the bit that really takes the biscuit. They've been camped out overnight to ensure they are first through the doors, yet as soon as they reach aisle one they see their neighbours George and Pat and start to have a bloody long conversation in the middle of the aisle! Both their trolleys have blocked aisle one completely. It then becomes like the M25 motorway on a bad day, as trolley after trolley start to stack up, unable to get through. People take a detour down aisle three to then come back up aisle two, but because everyone's got the same idea, this aisle gets blocked solid as well. Now comes the best bit. Maud looks around and then says to Pat,

"My it's busy today."

AAAARRGHHHH!!!!!!

Anyway, back to my blood test. I take my number

and I'm number 125. I reckon this number reflects the age I'll be by the time I'm called for my turn.

As the receptionist gave me my number she asked, "Have you fasted?"

I totally misheard what she said, what with all the chatting in the background about bombs and rationing.

"No I can't smell anything," I answered.

"What?" she said looking confused.

"No I haven't farted," I said, "Some old duffer's probably crapped themselves."

She laughed and replied, "I said fasted. Let me explain it easier. Have you had to starve before your blood test today?"

"Bloody hell, I'm sorry," I said in embarrassment. "No, it's a normal test with no starving involved at all."

I felt a right tit. Better sit down quick before anything else happens.

One hundred and twenty five years later I was called. I went into the room and there were six of us all having our bloods done at the same time. It was like a conveyor belt. I must point out that there were six nurses taking the bloods not one, otherwise I would've had to wait another few years.

I don't know how the nurses do this every minute of every day. It looked a pretty boring routine if you ask me. Sticking needles into veins and then saying the immortal phrase, "Just a little sharp scratch."

Now if I were a nurse I'd have a few more phrases to say every time the needle was about to go in. I would liven things up a bit.

I'd start off gentle and say something like this,

"It will feel like a little bee sting," or "Just a small prick."

Then I'd turn the screw.

"This is going to bloody hurt," or "It's going to feel like I've stabbed your arm repeatedly with a cocktail stick."

I'd save the best for last.

"It's funny. Yesterday I did a normal routine blood test, but because I got the wrong vein the person bled to death. Shame really, because he was such a nice bloke."

My blood test was done and off it went to the specialist ready for my appointment next week.

I also had to have a full body CT scan before my first check up. This was arranged one week before my appointment. The CT scanner is an excellent piece of medical equipment. It checks the whole body to make sure the cancer hasn't spread anywhere else. Knowing I was having the scan and numerous blood tests really helped to build up my confidence. The NHS were really looking after me and doing their utmost to make sure I stayed fit and healthy. As far as I was concerned, the more blood tests the better. Christ, I'd had more pricks than a rent boy in the last three months or so, but I don't care. It's well worth it.

I arrived at the x-ray department and was directed to a small cubicle where I had to take all my clothes off, apart from my pants and socks. I then had to put on the infamous NHS gown again. Oh how I enjoyed our reunion. How I'd missed you old friend. However, this time I wouldn't make the same mistake of not doing the bottom ties up.

A few hours before the scan I had to drink some liquid. This would show up the insides of my body much better when the scan is being performed. Also, I wasn't allowed to eat anything from when I woke up that morning.

The liquid can be mixed with squash to make it go down easier. I opted for Kia Ora orange squash as I feel this has a far superior taste over its rivals. Oh, and I used to love their advert on the television.

I wasn't allowed to drink the liquid all in one go. No, I had to drink a certain amount every half hour over a two-hour period until it was all finished. It bloody tasted fabulous. It had a twist of aniseed about it and tasted exactly like Pernod.

Once I'd put on the gown, I then had to wait in the main reception area of the x-ray department. My clothes were folded neatly and placed in a little shopping basket that the NHS provided. I looked a right wally as I made my way from the cubicle to reception, swinging the little basket in one hand, whilst the other made sure my gown wouldn't suddenly open to reveal my Superman pants. As I sat down the gown rode up slightly to reveal my Spiderman socks. What a picture. A grown man in an ill fitting gown, carrying a petite little shopping basket and showing off his extensive range of super hero accessories.

I was bursting for a pee, but I couldn't go as they like you to have a full bladder when the scan is done. It's terrible really. Here I was desperate for a slash, yet only hours earlier I had to drink about two pints of Kia Ora mixed with Pernod. Surely to God they know I would need a pee after drinking that amount of fluid. The torturing bastards!

Twenty minutes later the radiographer called me into the CT room.

I scanned my eyes around the room until they became fixed on the CT scanner machine. I'd seen them before on Casualty and Holby City, but it wasn't until I saw the bloody thing in the flesh that I thought,

"Bloody hell. Am I going to fit in there?"

Basically, I had to lay down flat on a cushioned bed, rectangular in shape. Well it's hardly likely to be triangular is it? The CT machine worked like this. The bed moves back and forth through a tunnel where above me pictures are taken of various parts of my body. Easy really. However, I didn't like the look of the tunnel. It looked bloody small and narrow. How on earth was I going to fit through this tunnel? Christ, my gut would have trouble getting through the Dartford tunnel let alone this one! I was going to get jammed in solid, unable to move. The fire brigade would turn up and cut open the CT scanner with their mechanical gear. I'd have broken the only scanner in the area and I'd have to pay the NHS a quid a week for the next forty thousand years to replace it. Please God let the tunnel actually be bigger than I imagine.

The radiographer suddenly interrupted my thoughts.

"Have you ever been in one of these before?" he said.

"Yeah of course," I thought to myself sarcastically, "There's one of these on Clacton Pier and I ride it every week!"

What do you reckon pal. Read my notes will you and you will clearly see this is my first time. However, I politely replied, "No, I'm a CT virgin."

"Right Mr Couchman. Lie back on the bed and place your arms behind your head and tuck your elbows in to avoid catching them on the sides of the tunnel" said the radiographer.

Bloody hell, the tunnel is going to rip my arms off before it wedges me in. I can see it now. The bad news will be that the cancer has spread to the bones in my arms, but hey there's some good news. At least the tunnel ripped my sodding arms off before the cancer could spread any further!

He continued,

"As you enter the tunnel please listen to the instructions and carry them out. It's important you do what the recorded voice tells you."

Bloody hell, there's a lot to take in and there's a lot to worry about. At least I was allowed to keep the gown on and not have to worry about the fire brigade seeing my Clark Kent briefs.

I lay down and the radiographer left the room to start up the machine.

There was a lot of noise as the machine started up and suddenly I was moving backwards and heading for the tunnel. Phew! I made it. Surprisingly the tunnel was a lot bigger inside. There was plenty of room and my arms felt safe. Thank the lord.

As I went into the tunnel, all I could hear at this point was a noise that sounded like something revolving very quickly. I looked up and above me I could see part of the machine going round like the clappers. This must be the part of the machine that takes the pictures I thought. I smiled and gave a thumbs up. This was immediately followed by a bollocking from the radiographer.

I wonder if it's like the white knuckle rides at theme parks where you rush off the ride as quick as you can, just so you can see the photos of you looking shit scared as you've looped the loop several times.

Suddenly my thoughts were interrupted by a female voice. It wasn't the radiographer because he was a bloke, although he was wearing black eyeliner and mascara. I think he was a Goth, as I overheard him talking earlier about sacrificing a goat on the next full moon.

Then I twigged. It was a computerised voice, the one the radiographer told me to listen to carefully. The voice said, "Breathe in and hold."

I did as I was told. I didn't want to annoy a computerised female. Crikey, she could laser my dick off in an instant if I pissed her about! Who knows what power she holds in this hospital.

I held my breath and waited...

Bloody hell woman, when can I breathe out? It's taking forever. I was just about to explode when she said, "And breathe."

This scan is supposed to be for my benefit, yet the bloody thing nearly killed me because I had to hold my breath for all eternity!

I wish I listened more to my swimming instructor at school. Everyone else listened to the instructor's tips on how to hold one's breath for a long time, yet I was just pissing in the water. "Don't you mean pissing about in the water?" I hear you cry. No, just pissing.

I didn't just have to hold my breath once. Try five more times. Each time I got redder and redder like a tomato until she finally said those words of relief, "And breathe."

The bloody robotic, futuristic slag of a bitch! I swear I saw the radiographer crying tears of laughter every time I had to breathe in. I hope his sodding mascara runs, the Gothic twat.

After about five minutes it was all over. The pictures, like my bloods, would be sent off to the specialist ready for next week's appointment.

I exited the room, got changed and went to collect the photo of my thumbs up. I also got a little trophy that had a plaque saying, "I survived the CT scanner!"

Of course I'm joking, but they should do this you know. It felt like a bloody roller coaster of a ride and I only just survived it!

The day of reckoning had dawned. Time for my first proper check up. My appointment was mid-afternoon. I got up, had breakfast and then it was off into the shower to make sure I was clean and fresh for when Doc inspected my solitary knacker.

I'd given up on my usual shower gel range and I tried a new range instead. This shower gel contained mango chutney and essence of poppadum. I brought it off some Indian fellow from the local market. Again I chose the worst product going. My nob smelt like I'd dipped it in a chicken korma.

I wish my appointment were in the morning like my previous ones. I could get it out the way quickly and sod off back home in time for Loose Women on ITV. I was going to miss it now. It's just not fair!

Was I nervous? Yeah a little I suppose. There's always going to be a small seed of doubt in my mind, even with all the positive vibes I had been experiencing. I defy anyone going for their first cancer check up not to experience some kind of nerves. However, the main thing was not to let the negative thoughts stray back into my mind. I achieved this by thinking back to what Mum and Dad had told me some weeks earlier.

Sarah and I arrived at the hospital and I reported in to reception.

We took a seat and the receptionist asked us to put it back. So we sat on some other seats and waited. I looked at the whiteboard on the wall and this listed all the clinics that were running today. It's always useful to look at this board, as this will tell you if your particular clinic is either running on time or is hours behind. I scanned my eyes across the board until I found the clinic I was under. Buggar. It was running an hour behind. I thought the receptionist was in a good mood when I spoke to her earlier.

Christ, by the time I get my nob out now, it's going to smell like a mutton vindaloo rather than a nice easygoing chicken korma.

I sat back and surveyed the waiting area. People of all different ages and backgrounds waited their turn. It was different to the other waiting rooms I had previously experienced. Before it was all old duffers, but this time they ranged from children as young as three to old duffers who had just received their telegram from the queen.

However, the message that this waiting room gave out became more apparent the more I looked around.

Cancer can hit anyone no matter what age, what colour and what religion. I bet everyone sitting here today thought that it could never happen to them. Just like I did. However, it has happened and we all sat here with one thing in common and with one question that needed answering. Have I still got cancer?

About fifty minutes later a nurse called out my name. At last it was my turn. Then another five people were also called. Bloody hell I thought. It must be a sodding line up. We've all got to stand in line and drop our pants, ready for the Doctor to feel each of us in turn. This would give a whole new meaning to the term "Privates on parade." Mind you, I felt sorry for the old girl whose name was called. I bet she didn't expect to have to get her lady garden out in front of all us men.

Luckily the line up never materialised. We all had to take another seat in a corridor and wait to be called again, but this time it would be to the Doctor's private room.

Half an hour later it was my turn. Sarah came in with me this time. I didn't want her to, but she wanted to see the Doctors face when I presented my mutton vindaloo.

Whilst in the room we didn't say a word to each other. I think Sarah was more nervous than I was. She was biting her nails and nervously playing with her hair. The room was quite small and it had a sliding door separating it from another room. This was probably where Doc sat and wrote out his notes.

The Doctor or Oncologist as he is better known, slid open the door and walked in. It wasn't the specialist that I had seen before and was expecting. Shame, I was looking forward to seeing him again. Never mind though, this bloke is an expert as well. He greeted us pleasantly and shook my hand. I hope he'd bloody washed his hands, as he'd dealt with the old girl before me and earlier she was complaining of a pain in her fanny bone.

He got straight to the point and I appreciated this. No messing about.

"Well it's good news Mr Couchman," he said. "Your bloods and CT scan have come back all clear."

What relief. It surged through my whole body making me shiver and get goose bumps (and I nearly ejaculated!).

Sarah's body language also took on a whole new concept. She was no longer nervous with her shoulders slouching. Instead a big smile spread across her face and her body sat upright, glowing in excitement. I think she nearly had an orgasm as well.

"That's wonderful news Doc," I said. "Thanks ever so much."

"It's my pleasure," he answered. "This is one part of my job that I really enjoy."

Yeah okay Doc, but I bet the inspecting of womens knockers and their fannies must be high on your list as well?

"I need to inspect your privates now Mr Couchman to make sure everything is ship shape," Doc said. "And I also want to take a look at your wound."

I lay down on the bed and pulled down my trousers and pants. I hope he likes curries. He rummaged down below, twiddling my bollock this way and that way. He didn't say anything about the aroma though.

He'd finished with my bollock and then he started to press down around my wound.

"How does that feel?" he asked.

"I'll be honest Doc, I can't really feel anything around my scar," I answered.

"No you probably won't," he replied. "This may be long lasting. Most people that have had an operation like you will experience a feeling of numbness around their scar. This may continue for a few years."

A few years indeed. To this day, seven whole years on, it is still slightly numb around my scar. It's a bloody weird feeling I can tell you.

He then started to press around my stomach area.

"Any pain when I press Mr Couchman?" he said.

"No fine," I answered just as my gut gave out a little grumble.

"You must be hungry," Doc said laughing." I think I'm going to pick up a curry on the way home tonight."

Bugger. The smell must have entered his nostrils and

encouraged his brain to want a curry. By this time I must have smelt like a little Indian fella who'd been cooking all night in the Star of Bengal takeaway.

"Right, all done now Mr Couchman," he said. "I'll see you every six months for the next three years and thereafter I'll see you each year until we reach the magic number five."

In cancer terms, reaching the fifth year and being cancer free is significant. This usually means no more check ups and a life of being healthy once more.

"At least I know I'm being looked after," I replied very pleased.

"We do our best," he answered.

And that was that. All finished. All over and done with for at least another six months. I was in remission and boy was I glad. I couldn't wait to tell everyone my good news. It no longer felt like my life was on hold. My life began again from the moment I left the hospital. The sky was blue and the warmth of the sun's rays hit my face. What a glorious day, a glorious day to be alive.

No regrets Mum and Dad had told me. You aren't wrong there. Life would be different now. I've had my wake up call and Christ do I feel awake. Except when I'm asleep of course.

Now I could go back to work and continue with my financial advisers course up in Leeds. Nothing can stop me now.

The drinks are on me!

Chapter 11
Silence isn't Golden

Finally, after months of Doctors appointments and hospital appointments, I was ready to go back to work. I was ready for anything the world could throw at me.

All the dates for my course had been set. There were no more appointments for at least another six months, so nothing could get in the way. There was no going back now.

I had already completed week 1 of the course prior to my operation, so I would be joining a new set of colleagues on week 2. I felt nervous beforehand. I would be a newcomer to the group because they had already spent the whole of week 1 together. How would I fit in? Would they accept me? I've seen Big Brother on the television loads of times. I've seen how difficult it is for new housemates that join the house a couple of weeks after everyone else. A tight knit community spirit has already been established and newcomers can upset the apple cart and become isolated. The course is no way like Big Brother, but hopefully you understand what I am rambling on about. Mind you, I suppose I could get evicted from the course if I decide to show everyone my bollock.

These questions kept replaying over and over again in my mind. However, I would very quickly find the answers to my questions when I arrived at the hotel in Leeds.

I travelled up to Leeds on the Sunday afternoon as the course started at 9.00am sharp. There was no way I was going to travel up on the Monday morning, as it can take around four and half hours to get to Leeds from my house.

I checked in at the hotel (the Hilton of all places) and went up to my room and unpacked. I think the bank chose the Hilton, because of my brush with fame when I did all the magazine and newspaper articles. They probably felt it only right that I receive the best of the best. Mind you, I would love to know what fame all my other colleagues had experienced, as they were all staying in the Hilton as well!

I deliberated about going down to the bar area to meet the others and introduce myself. The trouble was I was shit scared. I paced up and down my room thinking about what to do.

Scared indeed. I've been through worse crap. Here I am, a man who lost both parents to cancer when nineteen years of age and came through it. A man who has only just recently fought testicular cancer and won. How can I be scared? Pull yourself together you wimp.

They're only a bunch of human beings like me. We all work for the same company and we are all training to do the same job. Blimey, I haven't even met them yet and that's three things we have in common already!

The only thing I didn't have in common with the blokes was the correct number of bollocks. They've probably all got two, whereas I've only got the one. And then there are the women. They've got no bollocks. Mind you, if I performed my vagina trick that would soon put me on a par with the women. However, my pubes were still a mess so that was out of the question. This meant I was stuck in between with just the one.

I hadn't really thought like this before. I suppose I never had to. Since my operation I had been at home, surrounded by my close family and friends. However, this time it was different. I had never met these people. They were complete strangers and I didn't know anything about them. I felt different and I felt like a reject in society.

Of course when I thought about this scenario rationally, I realised that these strangers wouldn't have a clue that I only had one bollock. I mean it's not tattooed on my forehead. They had been told that I was coming on the course and that I'd been off sick for a few months, although testicular cancer had never been mentioned. However, I sensed that they would ask questions and fish for answers about my secret illness. If someone is given a little piece of information then they will always try and find out the rest of it at some stage. It's human nature to be nosy. I decided at this point that I wouldn't keep my cancer a secret from the group. Mind you, how the hell was I going to tell a bunch of complete strangers that I only had one bollock?

My emotional thoughts went into overdrive and I couldn't detract from the fact that I was different to everyone else.

Sure, I've told lots of people before that I had testicular cancer, but these were people that I know and love. You could argue that the people from Cancer Research UK, the magazines and the newspapers were complete strangers, yet I told them everything. This was different though, as I was raising awareness and this was something so important to me at that time. I was struggling to find a way of overcoming these emotional thoughts when it hit me. The magazines and the newspapers. Of course. How many strangers had read about my one bollock? Thousands I reckoned. Had I met each and every one of them? No. So what's so bad about complete strangers knowing I had testicular cancer? Nothing, as long as some good has come out of it I thought to myself.

I felt I had a duty back then to tell my story to help others. So why not now? If I keep telling my story now, then who knows, it may even help the blokes on the course have a better understanding of testicular cancer and how they should be checking themselves. Granted I was being a tad optimistic, as I hadn't even met them yet let alone spoken to them. Yet I was going to tell them in my first few sentences how to check their bollocks and become play dough connoisseurs. I didn't care as I had made up my mind. In that moment I made a promise that I would keep for the rest of my life. I would keep raising awareness of testicular cancer by telling my story to complete strangers. If they get offended then that's their problem. The magazine and newspaper articles had dried up, but my sodding mouth hadn't! What better way to get a message across than by word of mouth?

Confidence was now high and I was no longer scared. I was just about to go down to the bar when the phone in my room rang. I picked it up and on the other end was a bloke from the course. He introduced himself and said how about coming down for a drink and meeting everyone else. I really appreciated his call. Yes I had overcome my nerves and was no longer scared, but his call just reinforced the fact that I had nothing to worry about.

For someone to go out of their way, to find out which room I was in and to actually ask me to come down for a drink was fantastic. The questions how would I fit in and would they accept me had been answered. They had made the first move. They wanted to get to know me and accept me and by golly was I going to make sure I fitted in. They wouldn't forget me in a hurry I can tell you!

I went down to the bar and everyone was sitting around a couple of tables. A bloke got up and walked towards me with his hand outstretched and shook my hand. He was the one who had made the call.

"Nice to meet you Darren," he said, "I'm Nathan."

I exchanged pleasantries and told him that it was really good of him to invite me down. He introduced me to the others. There was an even split of men and women amongst the group. I wouldn't upset the even split, as I wasn't fully a man anymore and I was only half way to becoming a woman. Having one bollock, a pair of man tits and occasionally a fanny does place me in the middle somewhat.

As I walked towards them they all looked up and stopped talking.

"Everyone, this is Darren," Nathan said.

They responded with a mixture of hello and all right mate.

"Hi everyone," I answered. "I'm very pleased to meet you all and by the way I've only got one bollock."

Shit. What a fricking plonker! I know I was going to tell them about my testicular cancer quite early on, but not in my opening pleasantries.

They all looked at each other and were probably thinking, "Did he just say what I thought he said?"

There was a deathly silence.

"Right, sit down and I'll get you a pint," Nathan said trying to break the awkward silence.

However, my opening pleasantries had worked. Boy was I surprised. Everyone I met that night wanted to know more about my cancer. They were intrigued by my story, amazed by my story and touched by my story. For three hours I was constantly talking about my testicular cancer and about Mum and Dad to complete strangers.

Occasionally I asked questions about them, so as not to appear rude, but after answering them they quickly changed the subject back to me again. So here I was, sitting in a posh bar in a posh hotel raising awareness of testicular cancer. I never thought I would be doing this a few months earlier!

I didn't talk all doom and gloom though. I told them about the funny times also and how I'd been involved in magazines and newspapers. I told them how I used my sense of humour to help fight the cancer. The words brave and courageous kept cropping up in their conversations.

"No, not me," I replied. "My Mum and Dad were brave and courageous."

However, they still insisted in using these words to describe me. Of course it's flattering, but never once have I associated these words with myself. I didn't go through half the crap my Mum and Dad went through. I would never use these words to describe myself. It just doesn't feel right.

One of the other blokes called Gareth went up to the bar to get another round in. He turned round to us all and shouted, "Does anyone want some nuts?"

He then realised what he had said and was just about to apologise when I said smiling, "Cheers pal, but I'll just have the one thanks!"

Everyone laughed and in that instant I was confident the other housemates had accepted me. All I had to do now was keep up the good work.

Over the next few weeks the course was fantastic. Yes it was hard work, but I had some really good times whilst up in Leeds with my new friends and colleagues.

Throughout the long weeks ahead I would constantly crack jokes about my bollock or make up innuendos whenever I could.

This put everyone at ease about my illness and ensured no one would have to tread on eggshells around me.

A lot of the time my newfound friends would say normal things and not realise that this could be in some way connected to my cancer. Like every time someone would swear and say bollocks. I would quietly remind them that in front of me it's bollock. I always said this with a smile so they knew that I was only joking and not taking offence.

The way I dealt with my illness not only helped me, but helped the others in dealing with it also.

In a perverse kind of way I'm glad that God had mapped out my life in this particular way. If I hadn't been ill then I would never have come on this course and met some fantastic people. I've stayed in touch with two of the blokes (Nathan and Gareth) and to this day we still swap e-mails and texts. They both live in the cold part of England (up north) and are both fanatical Liverpool supporters. It was our love of football that connected us and it still does. Boy do I love sending them a text when Spurs beat Liverpool, although it's not that often. In fact I haven't sent that text for a while. Still, there's always hope. I even went to their weddings some years after our first meeting.

"What they married each other?" I hear you cry.

No, they married a couple of lovely ladies and now have gorgeous families of their own. I don't see a lot of them now because of the distance between us and also there's a great big wall to climb over that separates the north from the south. However, I know I am always welcome in their pastures.

So I've got two extra people who I can call my friends, yet I would never have met them had I not had testicular cancer. It's funny how good can come out of something so awful in the end. The only awful bit is they support the red part of scouse land. Shame really.

Part of being a financial adviser is advising people about life cover and critical illness cover. My training involved learning about these two areas in great depth and also how to talk to customers about having such cover. I was really enjoying the course and the social side of it as well. After a long hard day of learning, we'd often plonk ourselves in the bar to have a refreshing pint and then watch some football on the big screen.

So here I was, having gone through losing my parents and then fighting cancer myself, now learning to tell customers how important it is to have enough life and critical illness cover. To be honest, I didn't really need to learn the bit about talking to customers and persuading them to buy the cover. I could just call on my personal experience to convince others they needed it and to ensure their loved ones would be looked after financially.

Here's the stupid bit though. I didn't have any critical illness cover at the time I was diagnosed with cancer. Even losing my own parents to cancer didn't prompt me in to taking any out. Of course, once I was diagnosed it's then too late. I used to say to myself, "I won't need any cover as nothing will happen to me."

Also, I couldn't really afford the monthly premiums at the time. Oh how I look back and wished I done things differently. The benefit of hindsight can be so cruel. If I'd had critical illness cover then I may well have received a lump sum of money to help pay off my mortgage and to help with any other costs associated with everyday life. It's too late now. There's nothing I could do apart from tell others how important this cover is. To this day I am refused life cover and critical illness cover because of my medical history. It's so important to take this out when you are in the prime of your life and your health is good.

I suffered the financial strains when I was off work and believe me this is the last thing I wanted to worry about when I was fighting cancer. It just added to my stresses and it's fucking horrible. Look, I'm not trying to sell you life and critical illness cover just to earn some extra brownie points for the bank. I'm telling you, from my heart, to think strongly about it, otherwise you could well suffer the financial hardships I went through.

What happens to your family if you die? What happens if you become ill and cannot work anymore? How would you cope financially? These were some of the questions we discussed on the course. We discussed them till the cows came home. It didn't bother me dragging up the same old shit that I had just been through myself. I suppose I should've felt a little down talking about all these scenarios. But I didn't. The enjoyment of the course and the social side of it probably stopped me from getting upset or feeling down when I was talking about death and illness. The other plus point was that I was still raising awareness whilst I was talking about my experience.

However, what happened over the next few months I didn't expect. The course had finished, I had qualified as a financial adviser and I had passed my exams with flying colours.

I was ready to see customers for real instead of just role-playing with the other trainees.

I spent the next three weeks with another financial adviser called Richard (Dicky for short). He'd been doing the job for years and was very experienced and successful. His role was to shadow me and help me develop further and to make sure I was doing the job properly. He put a lot of effort into his job and was always at work before anyone else. Mind you, his wife's name is Dawn and his motto is, "Dicky is always up at the crack of Dawn!"

Now if a fanny in the morning is not an incentive to get up early, then I don't know what is. The lucky git!

So every minute of every day for the next three weeks I talked about investments, life cover and critical illness cover. Stone me, did I do well. Customers would say, "No we don't need any cover thank you."

That's fine I thought to myself, but listen to my story and maybe you will change your mind. And bugger me they did! Just by sharing my own experience with others, I managed to arrange a shed load of policies.

I had an advantage over every other financial adviser in the area. I'd been there and got the t-shirt (and now I'm writing the book). Who better to know what life is like when dealing with death and illness?

Every other adviser wanted to know how I sold so many of these policies, so I told them. I might as well make use of what I'd been through and at the same time I'm raising awareness of testicular cancer. I was killing two birds with one stone.

I even told the other advisers that they could use my story when talking to their customers and that way they would be raising awareness on my behalf. Soon everyone would get to know about the financial adviser with one bollock!

I spoke earlier about God mapping out my life in a particular way and how I'd made two good friends because of me being ill. Well this is another chapter in my life that may never have happened if I didn't have cancer. As I said earlier I was placed with an experienced adviser called Dicky. Now if I hadn't been ill I would have finished the course months earlier and would've probably been placed with another adviser altogether. This meant I would never have met Dicky had I not been ill. It's a good job God mapped out my life in this way, as seven years on he is my drinking partner and one of my best mates. He also proofread my story for me because he is quite intelligent and has a good grasp of grammar. Mind you, he did say there was too many swear words in the original draft. He said I used fuck and pissing too much. Oh shit, I've used them again. Pissing hell, I've just said shit. Fuck, I've just said pissing again! Anyway, I took his advice and I've only used them in moderation and when it felt right. Thanks for that Dicky me old fucker!

The three weeks with Dicky soon passed and then I was on my own. No one to shadow me or help me now. I'd worked really hard whilst I was with Dicky, but we had some bloody good laughs as well. There is one story that he still ribs me about today. It involves my tackle so I'm going to tell you about it. I'm sure a lot of blokes out there will be able to relate to what I am about to explain next. I needed to buy some condoms. At the time Sarah wasn't on the pill, as none of them would agree with her. She either came out in loads of spots or she put on weight. Until she found the right one we had to use good old Durex. I hated using them. Firstly it felt like I was shagging with a carrier bag on my nob and secondly I was too bloody embarrassed to buy them. The idea of buying condoms from the chemists scared me. It's like I'm saying to the till operator, "Yes I'm going to get a shag tonight," and then he or she looks me up and down and thinks, "Fuck me, a fat tosser like you can still get it." I'm embarrassed like thousands of other blokes that live on this planet. Mind you, the condoms do come in handy if I fancy a posh wank. I've often painted my nails a nice shade of red and pretended my hand belonged to some seedy hooker who gave hand relief for nowt.

According to statistics thousands of condoms are brought every day in this country. However, what the report doesn't say is that most of them are purchased from the vending machines that are located in the toilets of pubs and clubs. This way no one can see us buying our packet of three and we don't have to suffer a lot of awful embarrassment. However, the vending machine purchase was out of the question on this particular day.

I was working in a town called Bury St Edmunds and there wasn't a pub in sight. I needed some condoms. It was a Friday night, it was my birthday and I would be guaranteed a shag. Everyone else would have fish and chips tonight, but not Sarah and I. She wanted a battered sausage and one pickled egg! The only thing I could do was to pop into Boots and buy some. I asked Dicky's advice and he told me to stop being a wimp and just go and buy the things. As he was so confident I asked him to get them for me, but he said no. I think he was looking forward to seeing me queue up and buy them for myself. Cheers mate. We left work at five o'clock and off I went to Boots. Dicky waited outside. I didn't want him queuing up with me. Two blokes buying condoms together kind of sends out the wrong message. I found the condom shelf. Christ, there was so much choice compared to the vending machine. Mind you, the vending machine had one distinct advantage over the chemist. At least I could buy kebab flavoured ones from the Dog and Duck. As you know, I've got a nob the size of a Walnut Whip. This meant I would need to buy the smallest ones available. I opted for the straightforward ones, as Sarah has never liked the ribbed ones. She once had a dodgy portion of spare ribs from the Chinese and this put her off the taste for life. I told her that they don't actually taste of spare ribs and are meant for her pleasure instead, but when does she ever listen? There was one occasion when Sarah said she liked the taste of some flavoured condoms I had brought. The lights were off and it was pitch black. Foreplay began.

"I like these ones," she said seductively. "Reminds me of tuna and melted cheese."

"But I haven't put one on yet!" I replied. Great.

Anyway, back to the small condoms. I was shitting

myself enough about buying the bloody things, but to plonk the smallest ones down on the conveyor belt would really take the biscuit. I might just as well have a tattoo on my forehead saying, "I've got a small prick." I did consider buying the range that said "Hercules" to give the impression I was huge, but the sod would just fall off and then I wouldn't get my shag. There was no way I was going in bareback, not with Sarah being so bloody fertile. I picked up the small ones and made my way to the checkouts. Great, just my luck. A young blond bird manned the only checkout open. I thought of a plan. I decided to buy a large box of plasters and a large box of painkillers. I would then hide the box of condoms between the two larger boxes and just pray that the rest of the queue and the checkout girl doesn't notice them. Yes I know the checkout girl is going to have to pick up the box of jonnies and scan them, but I was hoping that the larger boxes would distract her gaze and she wouldn't even bat an eyelid at the box of plonkers. It was my turn to be served. I could see Dicky looking in through the window from outside and he was pissing himself laughing! The checkout girl picked up the plasters and scanned them. Next it was the painkillers. Now was the moment of truth. She picked up the condoms and went to scan them. She didn't even look down to see what she had in her hand. My plan was going like clockwork. I would leave Boots with my honour intact. I was just putting the two larger boxes into a bag when a problem arose. The condoms wouldn't scan. Shit! The checkout girl kept trying the barcode, but it was no use. I started to sweat and my face became red. Please just be a good girl and let me have them for free. £3 to Boots is nothing. But oh no, she did the worse thing possible. She turned to her colleague, who was about ten feet away and loudly announced, "How much are these petite Durex?"

The bitch! I'll bloody make sure I stock up on vending machine ones in the future. And I didn't get my shag either. I went to all that trouble and Sarah fancied cod and chips instead.

I was now a fully-fledged financial adviser. The good news was that I was based in the Clacton-on-Sea branch of the bank. This meant a five-minute drive to work and free parking along the sea front. Also I'd already worked at the Clacton branch as a cashier for five years, so I knew most of the staff and most of the customers too.

I had my own office on the first floor. Nice. This was the first time I'd ever had my own office. I've made it now I thought.

Each day worked like this. I'd see around five customers a day, with each appointment lasting around an hour. I'd then spend a further hour typing up a financial report for the customers. I would then pop this in the post to them. The report detailed what we had discussed and what I recommend they took out, for example an investment or some life cover. They would then come back a week later, after having read the report, and decide if they wanted to go ahead with any of my recommendations. I know it sounds boring, but I need to tell you this because it's relevant. Every second of my working day I would be talking in some way or another about dying and critical illnesses. This was seven hours a day, five days a week

However, after a few months or so I didn't feel right. I would come home from work and fall asleep before seven o'clock every evening. I wasn't very talkative towards my family and my whole body just felt knackered. This wasn't like me. I stopped playing with the kids and I lost interest in Sarah. I lost weight because my appetite had decreased. My sense of humour had almost disappeared. Sarah did notice the changes in me, but I put it down to the stresses of meeting high targets at work.

As the weeks passed things got worse. I would look

in the mirror and all I could see was a tired face. I'd pull my hair in frustration because I didn't know what the hell was wrong with me. On the way to work each morning I would feel sick to my stomach. There were many occasions that I actually vomited on my desk. Sometimes I even fell asleep in my chair, my head slumped forward onto the desk. Yet I carried on regardless. I didn't know what was happening. Was I ill again? Had my cancer returned? Soon I would find out.

On one particular day I suddenly realised what was causing all my problems. A customer phoned me and asked if she could come in that afternoon to discuss life and critical illness cover. I was my professional self and said, "Of course it's okay to come in."

However, inside I was hurting. I felt sick and I began to worry enormously. I vomited once more. My head was spinning and my brain was shouting, "No not again." What did it mean? I didn't know at this point.

The minutes ticked by and the customer was due in very soon, yet here I was shaking with fear. I went downstairs to get a drink from the coffee machine to try and calm my nerves down a bit. My manageress was at the machine.

"Darren," she said. "You've been different lately and you're not your usual self. What's up?"

And then, the very thing I didn't expect to happen, happened. My legs went weak, I fell to the floor and I cried uncontrollably.

I didn't stop crying for about an hour. I couldn't get up. My body and mind were so weak and fragile, although I did muster up enough power to punch the walls and doors a few times in frustration.

My manageress took me to my Doctors and for the first time in months I opened up. The words just flowed out.

"Talking about death and critical illness every second of every day is killing me inside," I said to the Doctor. "It's bringing back too many painful memories of Mum and Dad."

I'd suffered a breakdown. My body couldn't cope anymore and it had slowly shut itself down over the last few weeks. I hadn't told anyone about my fears, not even admitting it to myself. That may sound strange, but because I bottled everything up I was in fact stopping my brain from realising the truth. However, I'd got to a point where my body had suffered enough and I exploded. It was an immense relief to finally tell someone how I was feeling and it was also an immense relief to know that it wasn't cancer that was making me feel like I did. All my symptoms were stress related and led to my eventual breakdown.

I was put on anti-depressants immediately and the Doctor arranged for me to have some kind of therapy/ counselling. I'd only been back to work for six months, yet here I was having to take yet more time off.

After a couple of therapy sessions it soon became apparent why I had a problem talking about death and critical illness every day. It was nothing to do with my illness. No. I hadn't grieved properly for Mum and Dad and this was affecting me. The constant talk of death and critical illness was making me relive Mum and Dad's final days again. It was too much to bear. Christ, when they died I bloody cried my heart out, but soon after I had to be the strong one. My brother didn't take it very well, which is understandable. However, as I said earlier, there was a bungalow to look after and bills to pay. I threw myself into this and put my grieving to the back of my mind. It can take years for a loved one to start grieving properly and I was one of them.

I'd thought a lot about Mum and Dad's fight against cancer since my diagnosis and occasionally I cried for them. But I didn't greive. This is a whole different process. Crying isn't grieving. It takes a lot more than a few tears. However, my body was telling me to grieve properly for them, but I ignored it. I was fighting my cancer head on and I was using lots of humour to get me through it. I probably laughed more times than I cried during my fight. I was also busy with my campaign to raise awareness and then a few months later it was off to Leeds for my course. I was so busy over these few months. I should have grieved properly for my Mum and Dad years earlier, but I didn't. I should've cried a hell of a lot more tears and grieved for Mum and Dad whilst I fought my own cancer, but I didn't. My humour kept shining through and this put the grieving process on hold. However, although this was great, it was only prolonging what my body wanted to do. I wanted so much to beat my cancer and make them feel proud looking down from heaven. I didn't want them to see me moping around all the time feeling sorry for myself and crying every second of every day. I wanted them to see me laughing and smiling. However, I was doing the worst thing possible. Instead of just letting it all out and talking, I bottled it up.

I became confused. Looking back I can see what was happening. Part of my brain was telling me to grieve for Mum and Dad, but the other part was saying leave it. I was getting mixed messages. However, the constant talk of dying and illness at work soon took its toll. Yes I spoke about death and illness on my course, but because I enjoyed it so much this must have masked what I was feeling. And yes I talked about death and illness when I was selling a shed load of policies during my time with Dicky. But this was my first time seeing customers for real and the adrenaline was flowing. There was no time to think. Things started to go downhill when I was working on my own and after months of talking doom and gloom my body said, "Enough is enough." There's only so much your body can take isn't there? The simple fact was I should've grieved when I saw the tell tale signs, but I didn't and this led to my eventual breakdown.

Instead of bottling things up I should have talked to someone. Talking can achieve so much. Christ, I'd made a promise that I would talk to complete strangers about my own cancer, yet I couldn't talk to anyone about how I was feeling about Mum and Dad. Not even my family. I just wished I'd had the courage to open up to those close to me. Some good has come out of my breakdown though. I now know the tell tale signs of feeling depressed and I can open up before things spiral out of control. A lesson well learnt.

I never thought that I would have a breakdown. I was always full of positive vibes and my sense of humour always shone through. However, these were just masking the fact that I needed to grieve and I was using these to shield the real problem. If only I had spoken up earlier. The counselling sessions were really helpful and talking to my therapist was having a positive effect on my depression.

I talked in depth about Mum and Dad and about their fight against cancer. I'd come home from therapy and dig out all the old family photos and reminisce. I'd sit there laughing about the good old times and sometimes I would cry when things got too much. Sometimes I would cry in front of the therapist. I tried not to, but sometimes it just needs to come out and there's nothing you can do to stop it. However this was good, as I was no longer bottling up my feelings. It's better out than in.

Slowly, as each day passed, I grieved for Mum and Dad. Fuck it was hard, but it needed doing.

The weeks passed and I felt much better and I was crying less. At last I was getting somewhere and there was light at the end of the tunnel. That old feeling of being alive resurfaced and I started to play with the kids again. My appetite had returned. Not just for food, but for Sarah as well. Things were getting back to normal and

I had finally done my grieving.

I can't believe I put myself through all that shit and heartache just because I didn't talk. Blimey, I can talk for England normally, so why I just couldn't say what I felt is beyond me. Say what you feel for fucks sake! I know that now.

They say silence is golden, but in my case it wasn't. I finally went back to work about six months later.

During my therapy sessions I was put in touch with a bloke who had experienced testicular cancer and he'd set up a support help line over the telephone. The therapist said I might find it useful to have a chat with him. Not about Mum and Dad, but about me. I was surprised that my therapist suggested this, as I was dealing with my own cancer okay. However she said to give it a go and not to forget that I'd had cancer as well. Did it help? Yes it bloody did. To talk to someone who had been through the same illness was a Godsend. I told him all about the pain I had suffered after my operation and then I told him how I'd felt over the last few months. And guess what? He had experienced the same stuff as me. He could relate to every single word I said. I wasn't the only bloke in the world with one bollock. There are others out there. Someone exactly like me. Family and friends often said, "I know how you feel," but deep down they didn't know. They didn't have cancer and one bollock so how could they know how I felt? However, when this bloke said those words I knew he really meant it. He'd been through the same shit as me. I'm so glad I spoke to him. We even had a chat about something that had been bothering me so I decided to get it off my chest. A small lump, the size of a pea, had formed where my old bollock used to live. Quite rightly it had concerned me getting another lump, albeit a tiny one. It was a few more months until my next check up and to be honest I didn't want to see my own Doctor, as all confidence in him had been lost. So I told matey about it. Guess what? He had exactly the same thing happen to him. A small pea like lump had appeared where his old bollock used to hang. He had his checked out by his oncologist and it turned out to be a bit of scar tissue that can form after the operation. It's harmless and nothing to worry about he told me. I've still got the little lump now and it hasn't caused me any hassle. It's now a little memorial in my eyes. Every time I feel the little lump it reminds me of my long lost bollock.

Anyway, he had put my mind at rest. All this was achieved by talking. Yes, it's that word talking again. I can't stress enough the importance of it!

Just like me, this bloke had ensured something good had come out of his awful experience. We had two things in common. We both had one bollock and we were both telling others about our experience of testicular cancer. Silence is Golden. Bollock! Silence isn't golden. I've told lots of strangers about my cancer experience and some good has come out of it. I kept my mouth shut about my parents and look what happened. I rest my case. However, I'm not resting my mouth. No way. There's thousands more strangers I'd like to meet and tell them the story of my testicle.

Chapter 12
London Calling

I was always going to have the odd day when I felt down. Everyone does, so why should I be any different? It might be the stress of family life, the stress of work, or the loss of a family member. Who knows? I bet the person with the most positive vibes in the whole wide world has off days. No one can predict how anyone is going to feel on any given day. Sometimes you just need a little pick me up in life and thankfully I experienced some of these over the next year or so.

Some tremendous things happened that gave me a real boost and made me feel so good about myself.

It all stemmed from being a media volunteer for Cancer Research UK and DIPEX, the award winning health website. Yes I'm plugging the website, but what the hell. They deserve some free advertising.

To thank all the media volunteers (including me) who had given up their free time, the charities invited us to a few really top-notch events. The events were all held in London and the venues were in famous London buildings. I was so excited when I received my first invite.

Cancer Research UK invited me to a "Light up a Candle" service and it was to be held in St Pauls Cathedral. It was to celebrate all the good work done by Cancer Research UK. From my invite it sounded like it was going to be one hell of a grand event, especially when you consider the location and the venue.

The invite was for two people so I thought I'd better take Sarah. She had been through hell during my fight against cancer. Then there was my period of depression. She was always there for me during the shit times and she never ran away. There were many times when she had every right to walk away from me, but she didn't. She always stood by me through thick and thin. I can't thank Sarah enough and I am truly grateful for her loyalty and love.

Mind you, I had to take Sarah because everyone else I asked wasn't available, what with it being a weekday event.

I decided to wear my best suit and tie, as I reckoned the event was going to be well posh. Sarah dug out a really nice dress from my wardrobe. Yes my wardrobe. Bloody hell, I told you in chapter one that I like to get in touch with my feminine side. Don't you remember? Sarah liked my dress as she said she felt closer to me whilst wearing it. Each to their own I suppose. With hindsight I wished I never let her borrow the dress. She then took the pee and borrowed my high heels, tights, stockings and suspenders. Stone me darling; get your own next time. She didn't borrow the silky French knickers though. Why? Because I had them on.

I arranged for the dragon-in-law to drop the kids off to school and also to pick them up. It would be late by the time we got home.

We travelled by train and we arrived at London Liverpool Street in good time. Then we hopped on to the London Underground to make our way to St Pauls Cathedral.

There was absolutely no way I was going to attempt to drive up to London. I've done it before. It's too manic and chaotic and way too stressful for my liking. Sometimes it can take you ten minutes just to get out of a side road.

With the sheer volume of traffic in London it can take thirty minutes to an hour just to travel one mile.

I pity the poor people who have to learn to drive in this vast metropolis, although if they can get through this hellish city of traffic then driving anywhere else should be a doddle!

We had to leave early in the morning to make sure we arrived at the cathedral for ten o'clock. However this meant we would hit the morning rush hour on the tube network. Oh what pleasure it is to ride the London Underground during peak times. Don't get me wrong, it's a fantastic network of tracks and tunnels and it saves you an immense amount of time on your journey. But when it's crowded it's like nothing else on earth. Try Hell instead.

We waited patiently on the platform for the next tube train. It wasn't just Sarah and I though. There were hundreds of people waiting for the next train as well. We all jostled for position, trying to get as close as possible to the front of the throbbing crowd. There's a yellow warning line painted along the edge of the platform just to remind us not to step over this, otherwise we could fall to our deaths and be electrocuted or decapitated by a passing train. Our feet are dead level with the line. With the amount of jostling and pushing that was going on I'm surprised no one was pushed over the yellow line. Unless there's an invisible force field present to hold everyone back. Blimey, we can direct a missile to the front door of a terrorist's house so anything is possible.

As we waited for the train to arrive we are all saying the same prayer in our minds.

"Please let the doors of the carriage be right in front of me when the train stops."

A strong cool breeze starts to filter out from the dark tunnel to our right. Two dim lights start drawing closer towards us and a rumbling noise starts to build up. The train is coming. Everyone jostles again and we all move forward an extra centimetre, our toes now slightly over the yellow warning line. A few people seem to be falling forwards towards the track, but they miraculously regain their balance and straighten up again relieved. They are either very good tight ropewalkers, skilled in the art of balancing, or the force field saved them. It's bloody dangerous stepping over the warning line, but no one cares. We are all after the same thing and we desperately need it. A seat on the train. It's really rare to get a seat during rush hour, however people always get off at every station so there's bound to be some seats free. I just had to make sure the doors stopped right in front of me to ensure my bum would have a much needed rest.

The train slows down and I can see the doors on the carriage coming towards me. Slow down! You're going too fast! I calculate that it needs to slow down by another 10 miles per hour to ensure the doors finish up right in front of me. Blimey, how did I work that calculation out in such a short space of time? I didn't really, but it sounds good doesn't it!

Please stop Mr train driver, just about now. However, the bloody thing doesn't and I am looking at the middle part of the carriage. There are doors either side of me, but they are about two metres away. The commuters on this particular carriage are looking through the glass and are laughing at me. They know all about the door game and they knew I had lost. I don't travel on the underground that often. Perhaps four times a year? I'm a novice when it comes to the door game. I bet there are people out there who ride the underground every day and know exactly where to stand so they end up right in front of the doors. They've probably marked their position to perfection. Take ten paces to the left, walk forwards another four and make sure the poster of Harrods is directly in front. Bastards.

The train doors open and I grab Sarah's arm and we join the huge mass of people surging towards the small opening. I get elbowed in the face, kicked in the shins and I'm sure someone squeezed my bollock. There's no chance of a seat now. We cram ourselves into the carriage and we are now packed in really tight, like sardines in a tin. There's no room to breathe. I feel like I'm on the CT scanner again. I look around to see who's nicked my seat. All the seats are occupied by the city set. The businessman, the young stockbroker and the highflying single woman. Yet I can see a heavily pregnant woman standing, having trouble holding on to something as the train moves this way and that. There are seats on the train specifically located for the elderly, the mother with young children and the pregnant woman. However, I don't see any of these people occupying the seat. No, instead some young smug twat with red braces and a pin stripe suit is sitting in it reading the Financial Times. He doesn't even look up to see if anyone more deserving needs his seat. In fact no one looks up from their seats. Heads are bowed, eyes are closed and newspapers cover their faces. This is my seat and no one else is having it. That's the motto of the seat brigade. The signs that ask you to give up your seat for someone more deserving are ignored. They might as well say, "This seat is for the use of selfish bastards only."

I'm crammed up against a smart businessman who has his back to me, my groin area firmly wedged against his bum. It looks like we're ready for some gay love. I pray I don't get a hard on. Look, I'm not gay, but knowing my luck my old pecker will decide he wants to play regardless of the genre of the chosen subject.

I look across to Sarah and she is face to face with a lovely young looking brunette. Their tits are almost touching and their faces are only inches away from each other. As Sarah reaches out to grab the rail above to steady her, up goes the brunette's hand also and they accidentally touch. They smile at each other and apologise. It's fucking hot on the train, stifling in fact. Beads of sweat trickle down from their necks and nestle neatly amongst their jugs. Bloody hell, what am I writing here, a love story?

Their faces become closer still as the train jolts suddenly. Shit, they're going to kiss. I try not to look anymore as I can feel my todger starting to rise. The feel of the silky French knickers doesn't help either. Please don't become fully erect. It's no good though. The image created by Sarah and the brunette has done it. Up it stands, prodding the businessman's bum. Thanks girls. I try to retract a few inches, but it's no good. I'm jammed in tight. The train jolts violently and I move forward a couple of inches, my nob now prodding his bum with more vigour. Bloody marvellous isn't it. I couldn't move backwards, yet there is plenty of room to move forwards. The businessman looks round at me. I'm going to get a punch on the hooter, I'm sure of it. Instead he smiles at me, gives me a wink and hands me his business card and says we must do lunch sometime.

The train pulled in to St Pauls and off we got sweating like pigs. What an experience. People do this everyday to get to work. They must lose a couple of pounds a day sweating. It was like a sauna on that train and the worse bit of all was the horrible stench of BO. I must have counted twenty sweaty armpits as everyone reached upwards for the handrail.

I even saw one poor bugger's nose and mouth get jiggy with a wet armpit when we jolted suddenly. Thank God that journey is over, although we've got to do it all again on the return leg home.

We made our way towards St Pauls Cathedral. As we got nearer I noticed the front entrance had been roped off and all the tourists were not allowed in until after the service had finished. It would be temporarily closed to the public until that afternoon. There were a couple of burly security guards standing alongside the ropes and they were only allowing people in who had an invite. And for once that included me!

There were also a large number of photographers standing patiently behind the ropes. To their left were a large gathering of young girls and boys all looking rather excited. What were they waiting for? Oh yes of course. Did I forget to mention that the famous girly pop band Atomic Kitten would be present at the service? Sorry it slipped my mind. That's why all the photographers and the eager autograph hunters were here. Atomic Kitten weren't going to sing (to some people that was good news). They were the guests of honour when it came to lighting the candles to celebrate the good work of Cancer Research UK. Their roles, albeit bloody simple, were to basically carry the lighted candles a few metres and place them at the front of the congregation. Yes, lets call it a congregation. After all we are in a cathedral and it is a service.

Sarah and I walked towards the ropes where everyone was standing. They all probably thought, "Here comes another autograph hunter pushing their way to the front." But no, I wasn't an over excited fan. Instead I had in my hand an official invite and I bloody held it high above my head so that everybody could see it.

The security guards moved the ropes to one side to let us through and boy did I feel great! I held my head up high, my back was as straight as a ruler and I puffed out my chest with pride. Normally I would be standing the other side of the ropes, waiting for a quick photo and an autograph, but not today. I felt like I'd achieved something in life and to be part of something so big and grand, well it was fantastic. Here I was, a man with one bollock attending a glitzy service at one of London's most famous landmarks and Atomic Kitten were the guests of honour. Crikey, I even had the security guards move the ropes for me. To be honest I felt like a superstar.

Atomic Kitten weren't the only famous faces present. However, I'm not going to name drop, as this would steal the limelight away from the big attraction, Atomic Kitten. Actually I didn't know the names of the other famous people. They were the sort of famous people where I knew their face off the TV, yet I couldn't put a name to it. Who cares anyway? Like I said, Atomic Kitten were the main attraction and I was going to see them in the flesh. Hopefully lots of flesh. This was going to be one hell of a day to remember.

As we walked up the steps to the entrance I thought about turning round and waving to the cameras. I'd got caught up in the frenzy of it all. I was a superstar, albeit for about two minutes and I wanted to act the part. Just as I was about to turn around and wave, I misplaced my footing and fell arse over tit on the steps. What an idiot. My big moment had come and I decided to show off my bum to the cameras instead of my face. I dare not look round now, so I carried on up the remaining steps. I didn't want my face plastered all over the tabloids the next morning. What the hell am I on about? I'm a nobody. I'm not famous! The cameras weren't for my benefit. I definitely got carried away. Mind you, it's hard not to. The atmosphere screamed out glitz and glamour and I just wanted to be a small part of it. There's nothing wrong with that is there?

We took our seats in the cathedral and ten minutes later the service began. There were the normal speeches by representatives of Cancer Research UK and also speeches from people who had suffered from cancer and who had been helped immensely by the charity.

Twenty minutes into the service I noticed that the seat next to me was empty. It was at the end of the back row. Strange I thought. Every other seat was taken, so why should this one remain unoccupied. Suddenly, out of the blue, a bloke sat down next to me. He had a walkie-talkie in his hand and an earpiece in his right ear. "Who the hell are you pal?" I thought. You're a bit tooled up for a "Light up a Candle" service. Are you expecting trouble?

Then I heard him whisper, "The girls are ready."

He then gave a thumbs up sign to someone behind him. What did he mean the girls are ready? Was a line of dancing girls going to entertain us, or had someone ordered a shed load of strippers. Suddenly it became clear.

Atomic Kitten walked slowly forwards carrying the lighted candles. The bloke with the earpiece and walkie talkie was actually a member of Atomic Kitten's entourage and he had sat next to me. Of all the seats in the cathedral he actually sat next to me. Now there's a story to tell the grandchildren. Granted it's not a great story, but I haven't got many others, so this one will have to do for now.

Mind you, by the time I have any grandchildren Atomic Kitten will have disappeared from the radar altogether. In fact they seem to have disappeared from the public eye already as I write this book. Probably something to do with the fact that one of the girls is now pursuing a solo career. Shame really. I'd like to see them make a come back. Where are you girls? What are you doing? Please reform and make a man with one bollock very happy. In your own words, "You can make me whole again." Now that would be nice. A bloody miracle, yes. But it would be nice.

I fixed my glaze on the girls as they confidently strolled forwards. I counted the girls as they walked. One, then two, and then nothing. Where the hell was the third member of the band? Don't tell me they are changing the line up again. Kerry Katona has already left the band and she's doing Iceland adverts. Mind you, at least she gets 10% off her shopping. I forgot. She also won, "I'm A Celebrity, Get Me Out Of Here." She did really well on this show. I think she may have eaten a kangaroo's testicle. I can't remember. Someone did though. However, was it actually a kangaroo's testicle? It could have been my old useless one. No one would know would they? Mind you, it bloody looked like mine!

I never did find out why the third member of the band wasn't present. Perhaps she was ill or up the duff at the time.

I said earlier that this was a grand service, in a grand venue and that Sarah and I were both dolled up. Everybody else present were also dolled up. Well not everyone. Atomic Kitten must have received the wrong dress code. The two girls were wearing really tight jeans and tight tops and they were revealing quite a bit of their bellies and back.

"Bloody hell," said Sarah. "If I've made the effort then surely they could have done the same."

Shut up moaning will you. I didn't answer Sarah and I didn't particularly care about what she had just said. This moment was one of the highlights of the service in my eyes. I was watching two of the fittest birds in modern day pop walking through St Pauls Cathedral, carrying lighted candles and wearing the tightest jeans in existence. Christ, did they have the prettiest arses I had ever seen. Apart from Sarah's of course. How many blokes can say they have seen that vision of paradise. Well apart from all the other blokes present who creaked their necks trying to get a better view. Thinking back to that moment I should've contacted the Guinness Book of Records, as I'm sure all the other blokes and I would have smashed the record for the highest number of erect penises in one room.

I could see all the women looking at the girls and then looking away in disgust as the light of the candles glistened along their most lovely curves.

I bet some of the older women wanted to scream, "This is a house of God."

Ladies you are quite correct. It is a house of God and it's only right we use it in the correct way.

"Hallelujah!" I cried. "Thank you God for creating Atomic Kitten and allowing them to show off large parts of their bodies in your gaff."

The girls put down the candles and off they went, quickly followed by the bloke sitting next to me.

A truly memorable service. A few more words were said and it was over. The whole thing had lasted about an hour. There was to be tea, coffee and sandwiches across the road in a large hall afterwards. This would be a chance for everyone to mingle and chat about the service and hopefully bump into Atomic Kitten. I really wanted to meet them and tell them what an impact they had on the service as well as my nob.

We left St Pauls and walked down the steps. The photographers and the excited mass of spotty kids were still waiting outside. I didn't wave. I just concentrated on the steps and made sure I didn't suffer a Groundhog Day and fall arse over tit again.

We arrived at the hall and I immediately made a beeline for the rolls. I looked around, but alas Atomic Kitten were nowhere to be seen. In fact I didn't see any of the other famous people either. They've all probably been ushered to a private room for celebs only. At least I know where I stand now with regards to my celebrity status. Stuck in a room full of egg rolls and crappy vol-au-vonts, whilst the A listers tuck into caviar and cucumber sandwiches.

It was pretty crowded in the room and after about thirty minutes we decided to leave. Sarah needed some air and went outside to use her inhaler, as she's asthmatic. I didn't know she was asthmatic until a month after we had started going out. I knew she got breathless during sex, but I just thought I was a stallion and had knackered her out!

Sarah also wanted to hit the shops in Oxford Street and Regent Street whilst we were up in London, so off we went.

I must point out that it was a bloody good service and it really highlighted the important work that Cancer Research UK does every day. I thank them for making Sarah and I part of such a wonderful day. However, this wonderful day ended on a sour note. I took Sarah to Soho (the seedy part of London) and told her this was the best place for some serious shopping. What she didn't have in mind was a gimp mask, some handcuffs and a large leather whip. How was I to know she wanted some new jeans and a top?

Another event that we both attended was one organised by DIPEX, the award winning health website. How many plugs is that now?

The event was in another grand venue within the walls of London. It was organised to thank everyone who had helped in setting up the website, including the media volunteers like myself. It was to be held in the House of Commons of all places. Very posh indeed. The start time was eight o'clock in the evening.

It was on the day before Valentine's Day, so I decided we'd make a couple of days out of it and stay in a nice hotel. We wouldn't have to rush off home. We could relax, eat out at nice restaurants, shop until we drop and perhaps take in a show. Sarah deserved a treat, so I told her about my plan to stay in London for a couple of days.

"You're just after a shag aren't you?" she replied.

How bloody dare you I thought! This was my way of thanking her for all the times she had stood by me. The bloody cheek. Mind you, if I get her pissed at Pizza Hut I should be game on…

I couldn't book a hotel near the House of Commons, as they were all full up with MP's and hookers. Now before I get done for slander, I must point out that there was a hookers convention being held in central London that day. It was sheer coincidence that so many were booked in the same hotel where lots of MP's stayed whilst working late on a new referendum. It was so busy; I even heard that some of them had to share rooms.

Instead I had to book a hotel some twenty minutes away by tube.

We arrived at the entrance to the House of Commons and bloody hell security was high. Mind you, it had to be what with all the crap going on in the world. I flashed my invite, but this time it wasn't to some burly security guards. This time it was two policemen carrying sub machine guns. There were no photographers either. They were probably camped outside a nearby hotel hoping to catch the picture that would sell a thousand newspapers the next day with the headline "MP works extra hard during the night."

We made our way to another door and again the security was high. However, this time Sarah had her bag searched. I just hope she hasn't brought along her dildo that's shaped like a Magnum 44, otherwise we will be in the shit. Thankfully she didn't.

We then made our way through grand corridors furnished with wonderful paintings and ornaments. Then we entered the main room where the do was being held. What a room! It was so lavish. There were magnificent chandeliers glinting in the light and many people were admiring the exquisite old paintings on the wall. Christ there was some money in this room.

The event started with a few words by the people of

DIPEX and that was that. All over in about fifteen minutes. They didn't want to bore us with hours of talking. No. This was a chance for all the contributors to mingle and let their hair down. DIPEX wanted to say thanks and they felt this was the best way to do it. I didn't argue.

We ate good food and we drank fine wine. Sarah and I walked through a door to the side of the room and we came across a balcony overlooking the River Thames. What a fantastic sight. The river was lit up as far as the eye could see, and I could just about make out Tower Bridge in all its majesty. Opposite, the London Eye was lit up and it looked spectacular. The river is a magnificent sight during the day, but at night it is something else. Here I was, in one of the grandest buildings in London, drinking wine and looking out across such wonderful views.

I was being spoilt and I loved every minute of it. I was experiencing something that some people will never get to do.

I'm glad we found the balcony early on in the evening, as later on we started feeling pretty pissed and the views may not have been as good with double vision! The wine was free and by God it was flowing.

We started to mingle and we found ourselves talking to a lovely couple that were exactly like us. He had suffered from testicular cancer also. And he only had one bollock as well. His name was Rob. His wife had been through a lot of emotional turmoil whilst he was fighting his cancer, but she had stood by him no matter what. Just like Sarah had done for me. It wasn't just Rob and I that had got something in common. The ladies shared a common interest as well. Rob and I chatted for hours about what life is like with cancer, what the future holds and about life with one bollock. Sarah chatted to Rob's wife and found that they had so much in common. They talked about the hard times and the good times. Sarah wasn't the only person in the world to feel like she did. Rob's wife felt the same too. Sarah later told me that she found it really helpful talking to someone who had been through the same experience. I think she found it a huge relief to finally speak to someone who could understand what it's like living with a loved one fighting cancer. At last she could get things off her chest that before she had been too afraid to talk about. She wasn't alone anymore.

We talked and we drank. We then talked some more and we drank some more. Suddenly the conversation became much ruder the more wine we drank. We were well pissed, but none of us gave a shit! DIPEX wanted us to enjoy ourselves and we weren't going to let them down.

We laughed as we talked about sex with only one bollock and we laughed when the ladies discussed the size of our nobs. I didn't care that Sarah had told them about my Walnut Whip. I was too pissed to take offence. I was having a whale of a time and I didn't want the evening to stop.

The previous event we attended was memorable, but this surpassed it by far. It didn't need famous people to make it big and grand. The room was full of ordinary people like me. Ordinary people with fantastic stories to tell and share. Ordinary people laughing and enjoying themselves. It was a sight to behold. We'd all had cancer, yet we could all laugh about it. I can honestly say that this was one of the best nights of my life.

However, the party had to stop at some point. We swapped phone numbers as we said our goodbyes and then we made our way back to our hotels. I listed him in my phone as "Rob one ball" and he put me in his phone as "Darren one ball". We'd only just met a few hours earlier, yet we were still having a laugh right to the end. Truly magnificent.

We got back to the hotel and climbed into bed. I turned

to Sarah and said "You got a lot off your chest tonight love, so how about getting your bra off it as well?"

But she was fast asleep. The wine had taken its toll. It didn't bother me though. I didn't need sex to cap off a wonderful evening. Besides it wasn't my birthday. I closed my eyes and started to dream about Atomic Kitten...

I'm ashamed to say that I didn't get in contact with Rob and his wife after the DIPEX event. We said about meeting up again and perhaps visiting each others homes and having a BBQ. I could use up all the excuses under the sun to explain why I didn't call or text him. He lived too far away, work's been hectic, life is so busy etc. Yes these excuses were valid, but it doesn't take long to make a phone call or send a text. The excuses were bullshit and deep down I knew it. I'd found someone I could talk to and laugh with about my cancer, yet I didn't make the effort to keep in touch. The odd text and the odd phone call would have been okay just to see how things were, yet I still couldn't find the time to do these simple tasks. I felt really awful that I hadn't made the effort. The trouble was there was nothing I could do about it. I'd changed my phone and somehow I'd lost Rob's number.

However, God dealt a hand that allowed me to meet up with Rob again at another event organised by DIPEX. This time it was at the Channel 4 studios in London.

No I wasn't going to record one of their famous "Top 100" programmes that they put on nearly every Saturday night. Although I was offered the opportunity to front "Top 100 things to do with one bollock." The trouble was we could only think of 99 things, so the show never got off the ground. For a full list of the 99 things one can do with ones nut, please send a self stamped addressed envelope to,

99 Top Things To Do With One Bollock,

1 Walnut Whip Street,
Bollocksville,
Nutshire.

It was held at the Channel 4 studios because the Channel 4 news presenter John Snow is the patron of DIPEX, the award winning health website. Another blatant plug.

The event was a chance for John Snow to say a few words about DIPEX and about the great strides they have taken in helping thousands of people each year. It was also a chance for him to meet the volunteers, like me, and thank them for their help in getting the website up and running.

Sarah didn't come with me this time, as she didn't fancy it. For starters it was during the day and there wouldn't be any free wine to go round. Instead Uncle Joe came with me as my guest. He said he knew exactly where the Channel 4 studios were situated. I said I'd heard all this crap before and had he forgotten that the last time I visited London with him, we got lost and I nearly had a wank in the wrong hospital.

However, this time he had performed a practice run a couple of days before the event. He had planned the journey in meticulous detail right up to the front doors of the building.

Fair enough I thought. He's gone to a lot of bother to ensure we don't get lost, so lets give him a chance.

He was true to his words. We arrived in plenty of time at the correct building. In fact he'd planned it so well we arrived a whole hour early and had to wait in reception admiring a huge great fish tank containing hundreds of different colour fish. I hope this was the right place and we hadn't strayed to the London Aquarium instead.

However, we were in the right place and I counted down the minutes until an hour ticked by. We were led upstairs and we took our seats in a large open planned area. There were only about thirty people in the room so it wasn't as big as the other events I had attended. The normal stuff happened. The people of DIPEX spoke a few words and then John Snow was introduced to us all. He walked to the centre of the room surrounded by our warm applause. I couldn't believe it. I'd seen John Snow on the news before, but here he was in the flesh.

His speech lasted about ten minutes. He praised DIPEX for the launch of the website and in particular he thanked the media volunteers for sharing their stories. All rightly deserved of course.

A representative of DIPEX then stood up and asked the media volunteers whether one of us wanted to come forward and tell our story. Everyone looked down. No one volunteered. A few awkward seconds of silence followed until I thought sod it, I'll do it. I said earlier that I wanted to keep talking about my testicular cancer and here was a perfect opportunity. I stepped up and everyone clapped, although I think they were claps of relief rather than in admiration for me.

So here I was again, standing up in front of complete strangers and telling them all about my fight against cancer. This time I was nervous though. Bloody hell, John Snow of all people was about to listen to my story. After a couple of minutes of talking I suddenly became more confident and I was really getting into the flow of it. After five minutes you couldn't shut me up. I'd kept my promise that I'd made some months previous of telling everyone I met about my one bollock, including the great John Snow.

Suddenly the woman from DIPEX started walking towards me. I think she wanted me to wrap things up. However I wasn't finished, so piss off will you darling? I haven't told John Snow about the time I thought God was a lady with huge knockers. Just as I was ready to talk about God's tits, the woman from DIPEX interrupted me and said, "Thank you very much Darren."

The cow! I'm sure John Snow would've loved to hear about how my shaven pubes affected my vagina trick.

I later found out that John Snow was on air for the lunchtime news and needed to get himself ready. Blimey, I nearly made him late. Now that would have been a great story to tell my grandchildren.

I walked back to my seat and this time I think the applause was in appreciation of my efforts. I had done it though. I'd told another load of complete strangers about my illness by the power of talking. I felt good and I felt proud.

The time had come for the usual tea, coffee and nibbles routine. I was drinking a refreshing cup of tea with Uncle Joe when out of the corner of my eye I could see John Snow. He'd finished the lunchtime bulletin and he was walking towards me. I turned around and there he was in front of me, smiling and holding out his hand. I shook it and prayed I wouldn't say something stupid. I think I said some thing like this,

"It's nice to meet you Mr Snow, I'm a really big fan of your work and I did the speech earlier about my one bollock."

Yep, I'd said the worst possible thing. What a twat. Why couldn't I just say hello and be done with it?

He thanked me for my earlier speech and also for the contribution I had made towards the website. I was in awe of him and I was bloody nervous. I didn't really know what to say next. Come on; think of something relevant and something topical. He's the king of current affairs. I was just about to say, "So John, I take it you've still got two bollocks," when luckily the woman from DIPEX came over and grabbed his arm, ready for him to meet someone else. Phew! What a lucky escape.

He said goodbye and my meeting with Mr John Snow

was now over. How surreal was that?

This famous man enters our homes each night to tell us about politics, the war on terrorism and the state of the Middle East. This man's knowledge of current affairs is immense. I could've chatted to him about Gordon Brown or the price of oil, yet I chose to tell him that I had one testicle. I bet he's never had a conversation like that before.

Then we all got a nice surprise. John Snow agreed to show us all around the studio where the Channel 4 news is filmed each day. I got to see how the cameras worked and where John Snow stands when he presents the news. It was great. How many people can say they have had a tour around John Snow's workplace? Not many.

Whilst I was mingling, I suddenly saw a familiar face. I couldn't believe it! It was Rob! We shook hands and it was just like before when I'd met him at the House of Commons. Hours of talking and hours of laughing. After the do we went and had a pint at a pub down the road. We were chatting and suddenly I found something out about Rob for which I was truly sorry. I could see it was affecting him when he spoke. He told me he supports West Ham and I was genuinely gutted for him. I reckon having testicular cancer is easier than supporting the Hammers!

Time flew and it was time to head home. It's funny really. Neither of us mentioned the fact that we hadn't kept in contact. I think we were both embarrassed to mention it. And I had the chance to ask for his phone number again, but I didn't. I couldn't admit to him that I had lost it could I. That would've looked terrible. God had given me another chance to keep in touch with Rob and still I blew it by not asking for his phone number. I should have been honest and just admitted that I lost it when I got a new phone. He wouldn't have been offended. He wasn't that sort of bloke. You're probably all thinking, "Hang on, he never contacted you either." Yes, that is true and he's probably feeling the same as me (hopefully he is).

Mum and Dad had told me, "No regrets." However, not keeping in touch with Rob is still one of my biggest regrets.

There haven't been anymore DIPEX events for a number of years now, so I blew the last chance I had of keeping in touch. You never know though, God might deal another hand and bring us together again. Mind you, she's probably pissed off with me seeing as I blew the last one.

I said at the start of this chapter that some things happened that were a real pick me up. That night in the House of Commons was top drawer. Don't get me wrong, the "Light up a Candle" service and meeting John Snow were great, but nothing can beat the night we all got pissed and laughed about our cancer. Although I've not kept in touch with Rob and his wife, at least I can say they helped in making one hell of a memorable evening. Something I will never forget.

Chapter 13
Fate

Was it fate? Was I given testicular cancer for a reason? As I've said before, I'm a firm believer in fate. So yes, I was given cancer for a reason.

Christ, since I was diagnosed with it I've achieved so much. Yes it's been bloody tough at times and of course I wish I hadn't got it. But I did and I've made damn sure lots of good things have come out of it. You have to make the most of things that come your way.

If I didn't have cancer I wouldn't have met Rob and his wife. Then there's Dicky, Gareth and Nathan from the bank. Because of cancer I now have three extra mates on my Christmas card list. I wouldn't have been able to get a hard on whilst perving over Atomic Kitten in St Pauls Cathedral. I wouldn't have got completely out of my tree in the House of Commons. I would never have met John Snow and had a tour of the Channel 4 news studio. I would never have met so many wonderful people during my fight. My fellow sufferers who showed such courage and dignity. The nurses and the Doctors with their expertise and compassion. Great people who should be so proud of the work they do. I wouldn't have met the wonderful people from Cancer Research UK and DIPEX. They helped me achieve what I wanted to do the most. I couldn't have done it without their help and support.

Lets talk about the future now. How do I feel now? Well I feel great. Writing this book has brought back lots of treasured memories for me, although some bad ones have cropped up also. I laughed when I relived my trips to London and I cried when I thought about dying. I'm a much stronger person than I was before and now I'm more open with others and myself. Leah and Charlie are now old enough and they know all about my testicular cancer. Yes they take the pee out of me, but I don't care. As long as I can still laugh about my one bollock, then I see no reason why others can't join in also. Mind you, Charlie keeps reminding me that he is the head of the house because he's got more bollocks than me. Cheeky little git! Up until recently my chocolate Labrador puppy even had more bollocks than me. However, there was no way I was going to let an animal have more testicles than me. My nine-year-old son is bad enough, but to let a dog have bragging rights would be a disaster. Before I got the vet to cut his balls off he used to bloody show them to me all the time. I'm sure he sensed that I was inferior to him in the bollocks department. He would lie on his back and proudly display them. I swear that sometimes he'd deliberately make sure I was about and then he would start licking his two balls. He'd look me straight in the eye and start gloating. I would try to give as good as I'd got, but there was no way I could reach my bollock with my tongue. He had a hold over me every time. That was until I gave the vet £150 to make me him feel less manly. Order now restored.

It's been seven years since my diagnosis and I don't mind admitting that the word cancer is still in my mind. Even though I've been given the all clear I'm still wary of any little lump. I still check myself regularly though. Every little backache, stomach ache, or headache triggers a slight fear in my mind. Is it just normal aches and pains or is it something worse. I defy anyone who has suffered from cancer not to become a bit of a hypochondriac. It's still a worry to me. Will my cancer return or have I had my fair share of it? I don't panic as much as I used to though. In the early days, when I received my first all clear, I used to cack myself if I got any pains or aches. I genuinely thought the cancer had come back. I used to dread the cancer returning and taking hold of my remaining bollock, although as I said earlier it's extremely unlikely to affect the other one. However, there was one day when I honestly thought my cancer had returned in my solitary bollock. I remember the day well. Four years had passed since my original diagnosis. I woke up that morning and went to roll out of bed. Suddenly this extreme pain hit me. I couldn't move. My bollock was experiencing some really serious discomfort. It was like someone wearing steel capped boots had kicked me very hard in my crown jewels. Ten minutes later and the pain was still evident. It just wouldn't go away. It was permanent. I pulled my pyjama bottoms down to have a look at my bollock. My sack looked like it was going to explode. My bollock was really swollen. It looked like I was hiding a tennis ball in my scrotum. Mind you, it felt like I had a tennis ball in my scrotum. I went to touch it, but the slightest touch meant more pain. I lay on my back. I was in absolute agony every time I moved. By now I was shouting and moaning in pain. Sarah woke up.

"What the hells all the racket?" she said.

"My fucking bollock," I replied, "It's hurting like hell and I can't move."

"I'll phone the Doctor," Sarah answered.

So downstairs she went and phoned the Doctor. All I could think of was that my cancer had returned and it wanted to eat up my last remaining testicle. However, I didn't dwell on the negatives like I did some years previous. The thoughts of, "Why me?" and "Shit, I'm going to die," were not even in my mind. The pain was too severe for me to sit and contemplate these questions.

As you know, I had experienced pain in my bollock and groin area before, however this was far worse. Sarah came back upstairs and said the emergency Doctor would see me straightaway. It was agony getting out of bed. Trying to put my trousers on was even worse. Tears rolled down my cheeks, such was the discomfort. I eventually made it to the car and Sarah drove me to the Doctor's. The Doctor was concerned and he made a phone call to the hospital. Five minutes later he finished his call.

"I want you to go to the hospital," he said. "They are the best equipped to deal with this scenario."

"What scenario?" I politely asked through gritted teeth.

"You've got what I believe to be a twisted testicle," he replied.

"A twisted testicle?" I answered very surprised. "How the hell did that happen?"

"It's quite common in men," he added (well it isn't going to affect a women is it Doc). "Your testicle can twist causing you very severe pain and discomfort."

"Well I suppose there's plenty of room down below for it to do a twist," I said. "In fact there's so much room it's probably done a triple salco followed by a double pike."

Ten out of ten for performance my solitary bollock, but now I need you to untwist and go back to normal.

Doc produced a huge needle and jabbed it hard into my thigh. He hoped that the injection would relax my muscles and hopefully allow my testicle to untwist and return to normal. He also gave me some painkillers. These helped immensely as I made my way to the hospital for further treatment. The injection worked a treat. By the time I reached the hospital the pain was less severe and I could walk much more freely. I was kept in the assessment unit for about seven hours though. They had to carefully monitor my condition. A twisted testicle can be very dangerous if not treated early. Luckily for me, Doc knew what it was and gave me the necessary treatment. Good man. Eight hours later I was home and pain free. Normal service resumed. Why can't my bloody bollocks just lead a normal and quiet life? Mind you, it bloody scared the shit out of me at the time.

Now I'm older and wiser and I know lots more about this awful disease. As time ticks on it does become a little easier each day. Although I have passed the five-year mark, I still see my oncologist every year. I don't have to, but he gave me the option and I took it. Just for peace of mind and reassurance. It's nice to know I'm still being looked after. If the cancer decides to return then at least they are going to spot it and do something about it. I read in the paper today that according to research the biggest thing people fear in this country is cancer. It affects many people and their families, so it's not hard to see why this came out on top. I worry about my kids health and what the future holds for them. What with Mum and Dad's cancer and mine, I suppose it's only natural to worry about whether cancer will strike again in my family. When the kids get any aches and pains, I tend to panic a little. There's a part of my brain saying, "Is it something serious," or "Is it just a minor ailment."

Two years ago my brain was 100% convinced that there was something seriously wrong with Leah. She hadn't been feeling well and had gone off her food. She constantly complained of stomach aches. Her weight plummeted alarmingly. Sarah and I were very concerned. After visiting the Doctor's she was immediately admitted to hospital. Test after test was done, but they couldn't find anything wrong or at least give us a diagnosis. It was bloody frustrating. They sent Leah home after a few days and gave her some antibiotics. They thought she had some kind of stomach bug. However, things got worse and her symptoms were still present. On one particular day her condition took a turn for the worse. She looked really ill and extremely pale. Something wasn't right. She was also visiting the toilet much more regularly. On one of these visits she screamed out in horror. Sarah and I rushed upstairs to be confronted by an extremely frightened nine year old. There were huge amounts of blood in her poo. I was now very scared. I phoned the hospital and they advised us to bring her in straightaway. Further tests were carried out over the next week or so. It's horrible seeing your own daughter go through such awful shit. The look on her face was of utter despair every time she saw the blood in her poo. It wasn't a pretty sight for a young girl to see. She was confused and very scared. Mind you, she was bloody brave about it all. Test after test followed, yet they still couldn't tell us what was wrong. I feared the worst and truly believed it was cancer doing this to her. I know all about the symptoms of bowel cancer and passing blood is one of them. Yes, bowel cancer is unlikely to hit a nine year old, but you never know with cancer. By now Leah was passing blood at least five times a day. Her weight dropped ever further. I was so scared at what might happen to her. I prayed over and over again. Please let it not be cancer. After a few more days the Doctor came to see us all. He said he now had a good idea of what might be making Leah so ill. I braced myself for bad news. Don't mention the word cancer. I won't be able to handle it. In fact let me have the cancer. I'm willing to die to let Leah have a decent life. The old parental instinct had kicked in.

He never mentioned cancer. Thank the Lord. My prayers had been answered. Relief swept through my entire body. So what's wrong then Doc? He then explained what was wrong. Leah had an irritable bowel disease called Ulcerative Colitis. Her colon was basically covered in ulcers. This was causing the bleeding every time she went to the toilet. Of course it's not nice for Leah to have this illness, but at least it wasn't the dreaded C word.

Leah was admitted to Great Ormond Street Hospital in London. She spent a few days there whilst they carried out yet more tests. You can't cure a condition like Ulcerative Colitis, but with the right medication it can be kept at bay for long periods of time. It's a lifetime condition. Yes she will have flare-ups every now and again, but at least she is alive and kicking and doing all the normal stuff that girls do. Like pissing me off with her backchat and getting lipstick on her bedroom carpet. Mind you, I wouldn't want it any other way. I still worry though about my kids, but fingers crossed cancer will never ever enter their lives. Right enough doom and gloom. I'm supposed to be talking about the future.

I hope my story has made you laugh like I did in the face of testicular cancer. I hope blokes are checking themselves regularly whilst reading my story, book in one hand, testicles in the other. If you're lucky then hopefully your testicles will be in your loved ones hands instead. Go on, ask your partner to have a feel.

The best place to check your bollocks is whilst you are in the bath or the shower. The warm water relaxes your scrotum and it's easier to have a good rummage around. Remember that I found my lump whilst in the bath.

Listed next is the best advice I can give you when checking your testicles.

- **Cradle the whole scrotum and testicles in the palm of your hand and feel the difference** between the testicles. One is almost always larger and lying lower. This is completely normal.

- Examine each testicle in turn, and then compare them with each other. Use both hands and gently roll each testicle between thumb and forefinger.

- Check for any lumps or swellings, as both testicles should be smooth except where the duct that carries sperm to the penis, the epididymis, runs. This lies along the top and back of the testicle and normally feels bumpy.

Take this advice on board. It could one day save your life. Each year there are around 1400 new cases of testicular cancer in the UK. It mainly affects men aged between 25 and 35, but it can happen in older and younger men also. Although it's not a common cancer, it's important to pick it up early. If diagnosed early, the cure rate is excellent, approaching 100%. Okay, so you could be left with one bollock, but don't despair. Remember there's always the choice of having a false one and in no way does having one bollock affect your sexual performance, unless you are already crap in the sack. Also, having just the one doesn't mean you will have less chance of fathering any children. The remaining testicle produces extra hormones to compensate for what has been lost. It worked for me didn't it? So if my story helps some bloke pluck up the courage to go and see his Doctor then it's all been worthwhile. Men are reluctant to talk about personal or what might be seen as embarrassing problems, but hopefully my story will make blokes see the lighter side of this topic and even have a laugh about their meat and two veg.

I really hope my story has shown you that there is

life after cancer. Life doesn't stop, it begins again. I do hope some good will come out of my story. I hope my story helps other cancer sufferers and their families grasp the positives and not the negatives. Even if they take just one thing from my story and say, "That's helped me," then I'll have achieved something. I want all the blokes who are shit scared to go to the Doctors to say, "Fuck it. What's the big deal about getting my nob out?"

I can now say I've done it. The last piece of my jigsaw about raising awareness. Or is it? To be honest I'll always be raising awareness of testicular cancer. I said earlier that I hope men are now more aware of testicular cancer. However, I'm taking no chances. So if you are a bloke and I bump into you one day, then beware. I'll be asking you if you check yourself regularly and more importantly do you know how to check yourself? Now ladies, you don't escape my clutches either. I'll be asking you if you check your fella's bollocks regularly and if not why not? Come on ladies. I'm sure your bloke will inspect your breasts in return. A fair deal don't you think. However, if he says the best way to check his testicles is with your tongue, then tell him it's utter bollocks!

There's nothing left to say now about my experience of having testicular cancer. I've said it all. Oh hang on. There's one more thing I need to say. If Santa Claus gives you any advice on looking for lumps, then don't listen to him. He only checks his sack once a year! That's not good. Now if Postman Pat wants a chat about looking for lumps, that's fine. He checks his sack daily!

Chapter 14
You've Only Got One Mum and Dad

Nearly finished. The final chapter. Time for the emotional stuff now. I said at the end of chapter 12 that meeting Rob and his wife in the House of Commons was something I will never forget. Well something else I will never forget is how my Mum and Dad lived with their cancer. Living with cancer. There are two sides to this issue. Firstly there is the person who is fighting cancer themselves and secondly there is the person who is watching someone else battle cancer. I've experienced both. I've shared with you my story of what it's like to have cancer, now I'll share with you what it's like to watch someone you love fight cancer. I'll also share with you what it's like to watch someone you love succumb to cancer. It's not nice and it's not pretty, but as I said in my introduction, it needs to be told.

I'll take you back some twenty years to when I was fourteen.

Dad picked my twin brother and I up from school. It seemed like any other normal day. We'd been to school, worked hard and then walked through the school gates at 3.15pm to go home. However, that's where the normality stopped. Dad never picks us up from school, so why today of all days?

Perhaps we were going to the shops to buy some

new trainers. Yes it must be that. Only the day before I was moaning to Mum that all my mates have got the new Nike trainers and that I must have a pair. It's vitally important, otherwise I'll get the pee taken out of me for wearing the old version. Then I'll no longer be part of the gang and will have to hang around with the swots instead. The only trouble is, Mum and Dad need to buy two pairs of trainers every time. A pair for me and a pair for bruv. Having twins proved to be very expensive for my parents.

We got into the car and off we went.

"Why have you picked us up today Dad?" I asked inquisitively.

"I'll tell you in a moment," Dad answered.

"Are we going to get some new trainers," my brother James asked.

"No," snapped Dad. "Just be quiet and I'll tell you in a minute."

Obviously no new trainers then. Bugger. I'd better start swotting up on crop rotation in the 20th century. With this knowledge I'd be easily accepted into the swots gang.

So what's up with Dad then? He's not normally like this.

The next ten minutes went by in complete silence. By now I was scared. Bloody hell, I was only fourteen. What's wrong for Christ sake? Why is Dad in a mood? Something's sodding happened. Is it Mum? Are my sisters okay? Nan's okay isn't she?

There was some serious negative shit flitting about in my young mind by now.

Suddenly Dad pulled over into a lay-by not far from

home. He turned the engine off and looked round at us sitting in the back. He went to say something. However nothing came out. No words, just tears. Lots of tears and sobs. I'd never seen Dad cry before and this started to freak me out. James looked really scared and went as white as a ghost.

"Dad, what's wrong," we both asked him time after time.

After a few minutes he composed himself, wiped away his tears and took a deep breath.

"It's your Mum," he replied, his voice trembling. "She's got cancer."

"Cancer," I said very surprised.

"Yes boys," Dad answered. "Your Mum's got breast cancer. I'm so sorry."

"But she's going to be okay isn't she?" James asked worryingly.

"Of course she is. She'll be fine," Dad said reassuringly.

Well that's all right then. If Dad said everything is going to be okay, then everything will be okay.
When I've fallen off my bike and cut my knee, Dad said everything would be okay. When I've had chicken pox or measles, Dad said everything would be fine. And guess what, everything did turn out okay, just like Dad said it would. So why should Mum having cancer be any different?

"When we get home, act as though nothing has

changed," Dad said to us both.

"Okay," we both replied in unison.

"Mum doesn't want sadness and tears, so just be your normal selves," Dad explained.

"Does Mum know you have told us?" I asked.

"Yes," he answered. "Mum wants you to know, but she wants you both to be her two strong boys and carry on regardless."

"Of course we will," I said.

Jesus Christ. I was taken aback with Dad's news. I'd heard of the word cancer, but to be honest I didn't really know much about it and how it can affect someone. Why would a fourteen year old have an in depth knowledge of breast cancer. My knowledge was cricket, football, and how to remove a girl's bra with one hand. Not bloody cancer. This wasn't on the curriculum at school.

How did I feel? How does a fourteen year old feel on hearing news like this? Well I'll be honest. I felt confused. Dad wouldn't tell us anymore, other than the fact Mum had breast cancer and now and again she would have to go to the Doctor's for some medicine. In his eyes that's all we needed to know. Quite frankly that's all I wanted to know. As long as I had Dad's reassurances then I'll be fine. Mind you, I was scared and shocked at the same time when Dad started crying. Scared, because I honestly thought he was going to say someone had died. And shocked when he started crying. This was a new experience for me. When he said Mum had cancer I was relieved in a way. No one had died and Mum had something I didn't have a clue about, so automatically my mind said, "So what's the fuss about then."

That's probably why I didn't cry when I walked in through the front door and saw Mum in the kitchen. Mum looked like Mum. In fact she hadn't changed an ounce from when I last saw her that morning, just before I left for school. She was getting tea ready and was whistling away to herself. Mum turned around when I walked into the kitchen and gave me one of her huge welcoming smiles. She didn't look like she had cancer. But then again I didn't have a clue how someone with cancer should look. I was young and naïve and my limited knowledge of cancer made me think,

"This is going to be easy. Mum will be okay in a couple of weeks."

Add my thoughts to Dad's reassurances of everything will be fine and together this combination made me think cancer was just another ailment people get from time to time. Like flu, or a cough and a cold. My young naïve mind had put cancer in the same bracket as a few snivels, aches and pains. You take medicine for a cough and Dad said Mum would be taking medicine for this cancer lark. So they must be similar then? A few spoonfuls of medicine and Mum will soon be as right as rain.

I now know how wrong I was, but looking back this naivety was a Godsend. I didn't know how ill Mum was at times. I didn't have a clue Mum's medicine was called radiotherapy and what side effects she suffered from. I didn't know cancer could kill you. Cancer is not like flu. You can't just swallow some medicine and get rid of it. You have to fight the bloody thing and fight hard. Again, I didn't have a clue how hard Mum was fighting. As far as I was concerned everything seemed normal. Dad said I had to act as though nothing had changed and I was doing just that. My brother and I were shielded from the truth and for that I am thankful. I don't think I could have handled it if I had known the truth and seen Mum's fight with my own eyes. I tell you what though; Mum hid her pain from us extremely well. Most days she looked fine and we'd still go on holidays, out for day trips, visiting relatives and out for meals. These events convinced me even more that this cancer lark was only a minor ailment. If Mum were really ill she wouldn't be able to do things like this. Again, I didn't have a clue. In the eyes of a fourteen year old this meant Mum was fine and dandy. Yes, Mum looked more tired than normal and she slept a lot, but then so does someone with flu. Nothing that I saw convinced me that cancer is a major illness.

A few months later Dad pulled James and I to one side and said,

"Mum's better now boys. The cancer has gone."

Okay, it had taken longer than I had imagined for Mum to get rid of the cancer, but hey, she's got rid of it. I was so pleased that Mum was finally better. Good old medicine. I knew it would be easy.

Three years then flew by and James and I celebrated our seventeenth birthdays. I'd left school and was working for a bank. I had a good job, good prospects and was regularly going out on the piss every Friday and Saturday. What a great life I had. Mum was fine; in fact she looked a picture of health. The word cancer hadn't been mentioned at all in those three years.

However, life is not a bed of roses.

A few months after my birthday I noticed Mum looking tired and withdrawn. She didn't go out as much and spent more time in bed than normal. Her whistling sounded sad and her huge welcoming smiles seemed an effort. Dad seemed distant also.

He took us to one side and said,

"Mum's cancer has come back I'm afraid."

"But she's going to be okay again isn't she?" James asked.

"I don't know boys," Dad replied.

There were no reassurances from Dad this time around. This scared me immensely.

I wasn't a naïve fourteen year old any more. I was seventeen and my short time in the bank had taught me lots about this bloody cancer lark. Part of my job in the bank was to help people deal with their loved one's accounts when they died. I'd heard many touching stories of how someone had fought hard against this awful disease, but ultimately lost their fight. I'd heard many stories of the terrible crap people went through in trying to beat their cancer. It was an education for me, so when Dad said Mum's cancer had returned I knew she would have a tough fight ahead of her. This time I was shit scared compared to three years earlier. This time I knew that Mum could die. This time I cried my eyes out. I didn't let Mum or Dad see me cry. No way. In front of them I tried to stay strong. Mum would be gutted if she knew it was affecting me. Again, I stuck to routine and normality. I went to work everyday as normal. When I came home I had my tea and went out with my mates. Fridays and Saturdays were still the same. Go clubbing and get pissed. However, inside I was hurting. I knew all about the crap that Mum would have to go through. I could see all the negative pictures taking shape in my mind. Getting pissed helped me blot out these awful images, however they soon returned when I was sober. That's why I kept myself busy. When I went out with my mates we talked about girls and football. We didn't talk about cancer. Going out was like an escape from it all. It's just a shame Mum couldn't escape from her awful nightmare.

Dad told us that Mum's cancer was more advanced and that her medicine this time would be chemotherapy. This had been mentioned many times by my customers and I knew what this could do to someone. Mum's fight had just been intensified by this news.

Dad couldn't hide the truth this time around, because he knew I had a good knowledge of cancer. Also I could see with my own eyes how bad things were for Mum. It was so different to three years ago. With the cancer spreading and Mum having chemo, well things were bound to be different than before.

I remember one occasion very well. I walked into Mum's bedroom and she was asleep on her bed. I then noticed small white lumps just below her throat around her neck. There were about five or six in number. I wondered what the hell they were. When Mum woke up I asked her. She could have lied and said they were nothing, but she didn't. Mum told the truth. They were cancerous lumps and they were spreading. Mum's chemo was now more regular. Instead of every four weeks it was now down to every two. This took its toll on Mum. She was sick every day and she was so weak. Sometimes so weak that she would be admitted in to hospital to be looked after. I remember visiting her one-day and she said she had got out of bed and fallen over onto her back. All because she was so weak. Mum showed me her bruises. She was black and blue all over and it was horrific to see. The chemo was affecting Mum's immune system as well. A slight cough or cold meant she suffered so much more than normal. Mum's long beautiful hair fell out also and she started to wear a wig. There was no way Mum wanted anyone to see her with no hair. She always looked immaculate and she wanted this to continue. It matched Mum's hair exactly and you would never have known it was a wig. It's not nice seeing your own mother go through such awful rigours each day. The more I saw each day, the more I learnt about how horrible this sodding cancer can be to so many people, including my Mum.

Dad was looking tired and he had lost weight. I took the odd day off work sometimes so I could stay at home to give him a much-needed break from looking after Mum. The cancer was taking its toll on him as well. It doesn't just affect the person who is fighting the cancer; it also affects the ones closest to that person. It must have been hard for Dad. Seeing someone you love so much going through such terrible crap. It's not nice. However, he was there for Mum every day. I truly believe the love between them grew ever stronger, all because of his care and devotion.

When Mum was given a break from her chemo she really perked up. Mind you it wasn't for long. She would go back to the hospital for another dose, just as her sickness and tiredness had ceased. However, she really took advantage of the good days. She would spend hours making herself look glamorous, combing her wig, applying the right amount of makeup and choosing the right outfit. Blimey, she was only going into town to do some shopping, but she didn't care. She deserved these days and she had every right to spend four hours getting ready. Mum knew that within a couple of days the chemo would start again and life would become hellish once more.

The good days Mum had convinced me she was getting better and that in the end she would be fine. Never ever did it cross my mind that Mum would die from cancer? She can't. She's my Mum and I need her. Mum will live to a ripe old age I'm sure.

Over the next two years Mum fought hard against her cancer. Some days were hard and some days were wonderful. Mum hated the chemo, but she knew she had to endure it to improve her chances.

One day Mum came home from hospital and said she wouldn't be having any more chemo. Excellent news I thought. This must mean Mum has won her battle with cancer and doesn't need any more treatment. Over the next few weeks Mum seemed so much brighter. She wasn't sick at all and her hair had started to grow back. Her whistling sounded happy again and her huge warm smiles returned. At last, my old Mum is coming back. Mum went out most days and partook in her hobby of shopping. Blimey she spent a few quid, but Dad didn't care. She had earned it. When Mum came home from shopping it was a joy to see her face so happy and vibrant. I was over the moon. Fuck off cancer; my Mum's been too strong for you. However, my joy would be short-lived.

The biggest truth had been kept from me. The one truth that I wish I had known. Mum's cancer was terminal. That's why the chemo had stopped. Mum wanted a quality of life in her final months and not have to endure any more crap from the chemo. Nothing more could be done. It's bloody weird though. The chemo stopped and Mum seemed so much better. Of course I now know why she seemed better. The side effects of the chemo had been removed from the equation. It's utter cruelty. There I was thinking Mum was getting better, when in fact the whole time the cancer had consumed her whole body and taken over.

Not knowing this one truth meant I wasn't prepared for when Mum died. I didn't know she was near death with each passing day.

It was Christmas 1992. Ten days to go until the big day. Everything in my eyes was perfect. The Christmas tree was beautifully decorated and the whole ceiling was covered in a mass of decorations. This year is going to be a cracker. The best yet. Mum's getting better and she deserves a big family Christmas. On this particular day Mum was due to go into a hospice for a much needed rest before Christmas. It also would give Dad a break and he could sort out everything in time for Christmas day. Like the food shopping and the last minute presents. Dad told me that Mum would be home in a few days time to celebrate the big day with us all. I had no reason to think anything different. That's what hospices are about aren't they? To give care and support to the cancer sufferer and their family. Christ, it can only be a good thing can't it? A much needed rest for Mum and a break for Dad.

An ambulance picked Mum up that morning and of course Dad went with her. I said goodbye to Mum and I told her that I'd come up and visit her later on that afternoon. If only I had known how different my day would turn out.

That was the last time I saw Mum alive. Christ, I can still picture the scene and see Mum's face give out the biggest most wonderful smile she had ever given me. I didn't see it at the time, but afterwards it became so clear. Mum knew it was the end for her, yet she made sure her final smile for me was the best one yet.

The news that Mum had gone was broken to me three hours later when a nurse from the hospice rung.

"Is someone with you Darren," the nurse asked.

"Yes." I replied, "My brother, sister and girlfriend."

We had all gathered together at the house and were ready to go and visit Mum, just like I had told her.

Anyway, why the hell does she want to know who is with me?

Then her words hit me like an express train. Mum had

gone. I couldn't believe it. She was getting better wasn't she? I hurled the phone to the floor and fell to my knees. I screamed out, "No."

James and my sister Lee started to panic.

"What's happened?" Lee asked.

"Mum's gone," I shouted, the tears now running down my face.

The next five minutes or so were utter chaos and confusion. Everyone was crying and shouting. My whole world had collapsed in the space of ten seconds. I felt so numb. I felt so utterly useless. How could Mum be dead? When she left that morning for the hospice it was only to go in for a rest, yet now she's fucking gone. My beautiful Mum gone. Anger now consumed me. I punched a hole in the kitchen door and I repeatedly punched the floor. Why? Why my Mum? She's only 56 years of age. She's too young to die. It can't be possible. I must have imagined the whole thing and it's all a big misunderstanding. I picked up the receiver and the nurse was still there. It wasn't a mistake, it was true. She said it would be best if we could all come up to the hospice to help support Dad, and if we wanted to we could see Mum. I phoned my other sister, Denise. It was awful hearing her cry down the phone.

I was scared to go. I couldn't face it. If I didn't see Mum then perhaps it wouldn't be true and she'll be home for Christmas. I went into Mum's bedroom and found her favourite cardigan. I clung to it ever so hard. I could smell Mum's perfume. I couldn't let go of it. Mum was with me.

The drive to the hospice seemed like an eternity. The whole time I just kept thinking, "It can't be."

When I get to the hospice I'm going to give Mum her cardigan and she will say thanks. It's all a bad dream isn't it? But it wasn't. We arrived at the hospice and immediately made our way into the family room where Dad was sitting. He looked so fragile and lost.

"She's gone," Dad said.

That's when I knew it wasn't a bad dream. Dad didn't say, "Everything is fine." We all ran over to him and cuddled him tightly; our tears now rolling down our cheeks and on to Dad's lap.

Dad was with Mum when she passed away and for that I am grateful. So many people die alone, but not Mum. Her biggest love was with her until the end. Dad said she didn't suffer, just quietly took her last breath and then she was gone. However, I was angry, but I didn't show it. I wanted to be there with Mum and hold her hand at the end. Why didn't Dad tell us the truth? Because he was protecting us. It's a parent's instinct. Any parent wants to protect their kids don't they? Most parents would die for their children. Something I'd discovered as a Dad when Leah was poorly.

I felt so sorry for Dad. His soul mate, his best friend, his wife, gone forever and there's nothing he can do about it. How's he going to cope? How does someone cope who has lost the closest thing to them? Jesus it's going to be hard for Dad, but I'll be there for him. A protective instinct then took over me. I've only got one parent now and boy am I going to do my hardest to look after him.

After about fifteen minutes the nurse came into the room and asked if we were ready to see Mum. I wasn't ready. I was shitting bricks. What would Mum look like? How would I react? I've never seen anyone dead before.
As I walked nearer towards Mum's room I felt sick. My stomach was doing somersaults.
The nurse opened the door and I could make out Mum

lying on the bed underneath the blankets. I started to cry again, as did my brother and sisters. Dad didn't cry. He was calm. He had to be for our sakes. I walked nearer and Mum looked like Mum. It was just like she was asleep. She looked very peaceful. In fact Mum looked beautiful. I held her hand. It was cold, but I didn't care. I looked at Mum and said,

"You're at peace now Mum. I love you."

I still half expected Mum to open her eyes, smile and say,

"Love you too."

I wanted Mum to speak those words so much, but of course this never happened. Mum was gone and I had to accept it, even though it was fucking hard. Mum wasn't coming home for Christmas.

That night at home was very difficult. Our home didn't feel right. Everywhere I went I was reminded of Mum. I missed her wonderful smile and her infectious whistling. I went to bed feeling emotionally drained and exhausted. I could see Dad in his bed across the hallway. He was sitting up watching TV, yet he had his arm around Mum's pillow and he was stroking it ever so gently. This cut me up big time. I got out of my bed and got into Dad's bed next to him. I wanted to be near him and Mum. We didn't say a word. We didn't have to. We both knew how each other were feeling. Dad stroked my head until I fell asleep.

I visited Mum everyday whilst she was in the Chapel of Rest.
Some people can't face seeing their loved ones in the Chapel of Rest. They don't want to remember them in

this way. However, I'm glad I did. Mum was Mum. She wasn't a different person. It also gave me the chance to talk to Mum about the good old days we had together. Just being there with Mum, holding her hand, talking, crying and laughing. Well it's something I will always cherish. On my last visit to Mum I gave her some photographs and a letter I had written to her. She could take these with her to heaven. That final visit was bloody hard. I didn't want to leave, because I knew this would be the last time I would see my beautiful Mum. It was heartbreaking. Saying goodbye for the last time was something I never wanted to go through again.

Mum's funeral was three days before Christmas Day. Going to Mum's funeral was one of the hardest things I've ever had to do. However, it was comforting to see so many family and friends present. I wrote a poem for Mum, but I was too upset to read it out. The vicar read it out on my behalf. I'll share it with you. Bear in mind I was only nineteen at the time and was going through some serious shit. I could've changed the words, but I haven't. It's exactly how I wrote it some fifteen years ago.

What can I say?
What a wonderful Mum.
Such a tragic waste,
This illness has done.

My Love for you is very strong,
A lovely lady who could do no wrong.
You filled my life with love and joy,
Please don't forget me, I'm still your little boy.

Though now you are gone,
I have to be strong,
You wouldn't want me to cry.
But I have many memories of such a lovely lady,
And each one brings a tear to my eye.

Every night your face appears to me,
Such lovely skin for all to see.
I want to reach out and hold you,
Share your pain and suffering with you.
But now your pain is no longer,
My love for you grows even stronger.

Believe me Mum you are not gone,
Your spirit in me still lives on.
But Mum there is something I will never forget,
You are the loveliest lady I have ever met.

My love for you is at its highest,
One day Mother and Son will be re-united.
But until that day I must carry on,
I hope my heart, like yours, is ever so strong.
When you look down from heaven above,
I feel your warm and friendly love.
You'll always make sure that I come to no harm,
Around my neck hangs your lucky charm.

I cry myself to sleep at night,
Thinking of you and your will to fight.
Many things to say, chances so few,
But all through what has happened,
I will always love you.

That's it. I hope you liked it.

I remember feeling really sorry for my Nan at the funeral. No parent should ever have to bury their own son or daughter, yet my Nan was doing that very thing. Nan looked crushed. It's not right. I can't imagine how she must have felt.

The day after Mum's funeral, Dad had to take my uncle back to London. I stayed at home on my own. I wanted some peace and quiet time to think of Mum. The only trouble was I got all the family photo albums out. Every picture of Mum I looked at upset me immensely. I wasn't thinking straight and I started to drink large amounts of lager and spirits. As I said earlier, getting pissed tends to block out the negatives. However, the lager and spirits didn't work this time. I was getting more and more upset until I decided enough was enough. I wanted to be with Mum. I phoned my girlfriend and told her that I wanted to die and be with Mum again.

It was a cry for help really. I wanted someone with me. Someone to hold me and someone to cry with me. I didn't really want to die. How selfish would that be to my family? Besides, I made a vow to look after Dad and I wanted to fulfil it. I sobered up later on and then realised how much grief I had put my girlfriend through. I couldn't apologise enough.

Christmas Day was hard. A time for merriment and a time for families and friends to share in many joyous occasions. Not my family though. I didn't celebrate Christmas that year. It just didn't feel right. Sure I opened my presents, but my heart wasn't in it. I felt robotic as I opened present after present. I didn't even realise what presents I had got. I didn't care. I was so fucking sad. I missed Mum so much. Then I saw the present I had wrapped up for Mum. Christ, I forgot some of Mum's presents were under the tree. Tears welled up and fell onto the present as I unwrapped it. Why couldn't you be here Mum?

I looked around the room in despair. Cards written by Mum were on the fireplace.

"Happy Christmas Son" and "To a loving Husband at Christmas" stood side by side.

They had to stay up. This meant Mum was still around, albeit in spirit.

I read Mum's words in my card every day and every

day I cried. Tears are hitting my writing pad as I write this now. Christ, it's a long time ago now, but it still hurts like hell. To see Mum's handwriting upset me. It's a strange feeling. Knowing my Mum actually wrote these words a few days before she died. They are so special. They are her final written words. I pictured her sitting at the table writing the cards a few days before. She's smiling and laughing as she writes. Now she can never write again. It's so sad.

That's enough of that Christmas. It hurts too much to write anymore about it.

Some days certain songs would play on the radio that were Mum's favourites. I'd sit and listen and picture Mum whistling away to the tune. I could've turned it off, but I didn't want to. For three to four minutes I could be with Mum again whilst the song played. I really found songs a good way of letting go of my grief. Some days I would bottle my feelings up, but as soon as a certain song played I would be in floods of tears. It's not all tears though. Some songs allow me to smile and remember the good times. All of us have that special song somewhere in our lives don't we?

A couple of days later something started to bother me. I couldn't shake it off. I tried to think of other things, but it wouldn't go away. It was about Dad. Mum's gone now and Dad is on his own. He's really down at the moment, but what about later on. Two years down the road he might want company again. What if he finds a new woman in his life? Surely to God he wouldn't want to replace Mum? Mum's the love of his life, not some other woman. This really cut me up, but I didn't say anything to Dad. Not yet anyway. It's still too early. If he does find a new woman later on then I'm going to make her life hell. I'll hate any woman that tries to replace my Mum. I know it sounds selfish, but that's how I felt. I'm sure I am not alone in having these thoughts.

However, I needn't have worried about this situation ever happening.

Over the next three weeks or so I noticed Dad wasn't looking right. He'd lost weight, he looked more tired than normal and he slept quite a lot.

I put it down to him missing Mum and that this was normal for someone who was grieving for his or her loved one.

However, on one particular night, the reasons as to why he didn't look right became all too clear.

I was awoken by Dad shouting out in pain. I got out of bed and went into his bedroom. He wasn't in there. The shouts were coming from the bathroom. I knocked on the door and asked him if he was okay. What a bloody stupid question. Course he wasn't okay. He opened the door and made his way back to his bed, where he promptly fell onto it knackered. Whatever had happened had ripped the shit out of him.

"Bloody hell Dad, what's up?" I asked.

"I'm passing blood when I pee," he replied in agony.

"Blimey Dad, that isn't right," I said now worried.

"I'll go and see the Doctor first thing," he answered.

"I'll take you," I said. "You're in no fit state to be driving."

He drifted off to sleep. The whole event had really drained him.

I went back to bed and kept thinking what was wrong with Dad. I didn't sleep at all that night. I was worried. I was supposed to be looking after Dad, yet here he was in severe pain. I wasn't doing my job very well was I?

The next day arrived. I didn't take Dad to the Doctor's after all. I had to call an ambulance instead. He was in severe pain and couldn't walk. He looked really ill. The whole situation cried out that something serious was up.

Dad and I arrived at casualty. He was transferred to a bed where a Doctor came to assess him. I asked if they could give Dad some strong painkillers to try and ease his discomfort. They duly obliged. We waited around for hours. Dad was still in some pain, but not as much as before. The Doctor eventually came back and said they were going to transfer Dad to a ward where they would carry out further tests to see what was wrong.

I was so focused on making sure Dad was okay, that it didn't even occur to me to phone my brother and sisters to let them know where Dad was.

When I did phone them I explained that my mind was elsewhere and that I was sorry for not telling them sooner. However, they were pissed off and rightly so. He's their Dad as well, not just mine.

After a couple of days of tests and scans the Doctors knew what was wrong with Dad. They told Dad in private whilst we weren't there. He broke the news to us all later on that day when we came to visit him.

He had cancer. Fucking cancer. Here we go again. Not only had it taken my Mum, it was now trying to take my Dad as well. I was gutted. All the emotions I had felt with Mum now resurfaced again. It was now Dad's turn to fight, however I'd be right there beside him every step of the way. Together we will win this fight. You're not taking my Dad as well you vicious fucking disease.

However, what Dad told me next I wasn't prepared for. His cancer was terminal. I hate that word terminal. It's so cold and final. Nothing could be done for Dad. At most he had a week left. Now hold on. How could it be terminal? He's only had the symptoms for a few days, so surely it's been caught early enough to be treated. But no. Dad told me he'd had the symptoms for about eight months, but he kept it quiet so as not to upset Mum or us. He said he was sorry, however I can see why he did it.

"Don't apologise," I said, "You did it for Mum and us."

Now that's what you call a cracking Dad and husband. Thinking of his family first in such dreadful circumstances. A credit to the union of fathers.

I knew what to expect over the next few days. I knew my Dad was going to die. Dad knew he was going to die. This awful scenario was so different to when Mum died. I didn't have a clue Mum was dying; yet with Dad I could plan things. I could tell him stuff that I'd do when he's gone. Like look after the garden and his precious tomatoes.

I could tell him, "I love you," and he would hear it. I could hold his hand and he could feel it. It still hurt though, knowing he was going to die. Every minute that ticked away meant he was nearer to death. How I wish time could have stood still that day.

Dad was smiling and laughing as we spoke. It's tragic to know that in a few days he would laugh no more. However, he knew he would be with Mum again very soon. This helped him and me immensely. No other woman would take Mum's place after all. Something I had dreaded. Of course I didn't want Dad to die. However, he was dying, but at least my Mum and Dad would be together again. I think Dad knew some months previous that he had cancer. He fought his battle in private. He hid the pain from Mum whilst she was battling her illness, yet as soon as Mum went, Dad gave up his fight. He wanted to die and be with his beloved wife once more. Soon that fateful day would arrive.

The next day I caught a glimpse of Dad waving to someone above his bed and he said,

"Not long now darling."

Was Mum here with Dad? Was she waiting for him so they could go to heaven hand in hand? I like to think so. I truly believe people see things just before they die. Perhaps a loved one, the tunnel with a light at the end, or miles upon miles of flower filled meadows. I hope I experience these when I eventually leave this world.

Dad's drugs and medicines were increased over the next couple of days, as his pain was getting worse. The drugs worked a bit, however he was completely out of it. He wasn't making sense when he spoke and he couldn't get comfortable on his bed because of the pain. It's soul destroying to see this happen to someone you love so much.

As a family we all agreed we wanted Dad to go into the same hospice as Mum. We all wanted him to spend his final few days in there. As you would expect, the care and treatment would be so much better than a bog standard hospital ward. He could die with dignity.

Unfortunately, although the wheels were put into motion, Dad died the day before he was due to go into the hospice. He was 57. He died five weeks after Mum. Again, like Mum, he was too young to die.

We were all with Dad when he took his final breath. We held his hands and cried. Dad knew we were all there with him, even though he was now slipping into a coma. I think he tried to say something just before he went, but he couldn't get any words out. His breathing became shallow and finally it stopped. Dad was in pain no more.

Although it hurt to watch him die, there was a sense of relief in me. He could now go to Mum. It has to be one of the worst things I have ever experienced though. Watching someone's life fading away in front of you. A life of fun, experience, knowledge and love. Snuffed out in an instant. God this is a fucking cruel world. I wouldn't wish this on my worst enemy.

I was empty and I was confused. I couldn't fathom out why Dad had gone as well. My head hurt like hell trying to think of an answer. However, my brain was not co-operating. The worst feeling I had was guilt. I'd promised to look after Dad, yet I've just watched him die right before my own eyes. I felt so bloody useless and a complete waste of space. I had one job to do and I blew it. I blamed myself. What if? Should I have done things different? Of course everyone said not to be so stupid and that I wasn't to blame. Rationally, I know they are right and I'm not to blame, but emotionally it's a different story. I can't detach myself from the blame. It's stuck with me forever.

Then I have to contend with the other type of guilt. I should have spent more time with Mum and Dad instead of going out with my mates or girlfriend. I should have helped more around the house rather then letting Mum and Dad do it all. I should have talked to them both more and told them I loved them everyday. There should have been more hugs as well. We could have had one final holiday together. I defy anyone who has lost someone close to them not to have these terrible feelings of guilt. However it's too late now. It's all ifs and buts.

My whole life had been ripped apart. To lose one parent is bad enough, but both within a five-week period is very hard to take. Why me? Why my Mum and Dad? It's just not fair.

Why couldn't the cancer happen to the scum of the

earth like murderers, rapists, or paedophiles? Why pick on two innocent, hard working, law abiding people? Is there a God out there? Yes I believe there is a God, but lets just say the almighty wasn't top of my Christmas card list. It's that age-old question. If there is a God, then why do these things happen? Why my family? Have I not been to church enough? Is it because I don't say a prayer every night?

As time goes on I've learnt to accept that God took Mum and Dad for a reason. God takes the good ones so that they can share their love and warmth with everyone else in heaven and make it a paradise. Yep, that's my theory. I still wish God hadn't taken them though.

I visited Dad in the Chapel of Rest also. I had to go through that awful task of saying goodbye for the final time. Something I said that I never wanted to go through again, yet just five weeks later it became a reality.

Dad's funeral was six weeks after Mum's. Attending two funerals in such a short space of time is bad enough, but when it's your own parents it's unbelievably tough. Again, I took comfort in the fact that so many family and friends turned out to give Dad a good send off. I also wrote a poem for Dad. Here it is.

What can I say?
What a wonderful Dad.
When you left this world,
I felt so sad.

You are now at peace and fast asleep
It's the way you wanted it to be.
You are now with Mum, together again,
In a way I am so pleased.

I was with you by your side,
Holding your hand when you sadly died.
My last words were I love you,
You looked at me and said them too.

Your spirit rose to the world above,
Once again to give Mum your love.
But my love for you will never die,
Believe me Dad, that love is high.

I will always remember those precious years,
Those special times bring a special tear.
This illness Dad, has not won,
It hasn't divided Father and Son.

With you Dad life was never sad,
Times were good, never bad.
Together we done so many things,
Your memories are with me as I wear your ring.

Times will be hard when you're not there,
I'll always miss your love and care.
I know you are happy up there with Mum,
But I'll make you proud to have had a son.

In the years to come I will never forget,
You are the best old boy that I have ever met.
But in all the things that I now do,
Remember Dad, I will always love you.

I hope you liked this poem too.

The hardest part in both funerals was watching Mum
and Dad's coffins moving slowly off into the background
as the curtain moved round. My view of their coffins
was getting smaller, until eventually I couldn't see them
any more. Their favourite songs were playing as this

happened. I was distraught. It's final now. Whilst the coffins were in my eye line Mum and Dad were still here with me. Once out of sight it was over. The end. The end of two wonderful lives.

Family and friends rallied around James and I. My sisters were married and had homes of their own. James and I agreed we would stay on in our home and run things together. Blimey we grew up fast. We had to. There were bills to pay and the house to look after. However, we only had to pick up the phone and a family member or friend would be round to help us. Sometimes it was to help us start the lawnmower or sort out how the central heating worked. Most of the time we just wanted someone to talk to. Family and friends are so important at a time like this, and none more so than our next door neighbours. They helped James and I immensely. Nothing was too much trouble for them and they always popped in each day to make sure everything was okay. People like that are rare commodities nowadays.

Running the house actually helped me take my mind off all the crap that had happened. Every day was tough still, but now I had responsibility. Housework and looking after the garden took priority. I promised Dad I would look after his precious tomatoes and I wasn't going to let him down. Of course it was weird not having them around. The house seemed empty. I'd cry when I came across photos or stumble across pieces of paper with their handwriting on. However, as time went on, smiles and laughter replaced my tears. I would try and remember silly little things like when was the last time we all sat in the garden together. Or what was the last programme we all watched together. Remembering these things helped. With each passing day, things got a little easier.

One thing I did struggle with was sorting out Mum and Dad's bedroom. It took me a whole year before I could sort it out. I suppose I turned their bedroom into a sort of shrine. Everything was left as it was. No one was allowed to move anything or touch anything. If the room remained exactly the same then it made it easier for me to remember them. Mum's hand creams and perfumes stood neatly on her dressing table. Dad's shoes were placed under the bed and his coat was hung on the back of the door. These items allowed me to reminisce. I could see Mum sitting at her dresser, combing her long beautiful hair. She then applies her hand cream and sprays her favourite perfume onto her wrist. I can smell it so clearly. Then Dad walks in, gives Mum a kiss and then promptly throws his shoes under the bed. Mum shakes her head in disapproval, as there is a cupboard in the hall for all the shoes. You see it's these memories I needed to keep alive and see everyday. My shrine made these things happen. However, as time went on, I realised I needed to move on and make the horrible decision of clearing out their things. It was horrible sorting through their clothes and deciding what to get rid of. I even tried most of Dad's things on, praying they would fit me so that I didn't have to get rid of them. However, they were miles too big and to be honest not my idea of fashion. Every time I put an item of clothing into the black bin bag, it felt like I was letting them down. Worst of all it felt like I was letting a piece of them go. However, it had to be done and the cancer charity shops would benefit. That's what Mum and Dad would have wanted.

A few weeks after Dad's funeral we scattered Mum and Dad's ashes together. In their memory we decided to have a bench and a rosebush at the crematorium. Somewhere I can visit and place flowers every birthday, Christmas, Mothers Day and Fathers Day. I also visit the crematorium on the anniversaries of their passing. The bench and rosebush are focal points that allow me to be close to my parents. I can sit on the bench and talk to Mum and Dad. I can place my flowers next to the rosebush. I always visit the crematorium on these special dates. I try my hardest not to miss any. Otherwise I feel like I'm letting them down. Of course there are times when it's impossible to go, like if I'm on holiday, but I know I will be forgiven for this. There have been times more recently that I have forgotten though. You know how it is. We all lead hectic lives. I feel really awful when I forget. I make sure I visit the next day with an extra big bunch of flowers. I stay a little longer as well. This is to say sorry to Mum and Dad and to try and make it up to them. I know it sounds silly, but it makes me feel better.

When we scattered their ashes this was something I would never have envisaged happening, but here we all were on a cold February day sending off Mum and Dad to heaven together. That's the important word, together. Nothing was going to keep my Mum and Dad apart. It was fate. It's strange to say it, but that fucking awful disease called cancer actually ensured they would be together again. Not apart, pining for each other, but together. Holding hands and sharing a cloud up in heaven. Don't get me wrong. I hate the disease called cancer. It took the two most precious people to me at that time.

I get really pissed off when people moan about their Mum and Dad or fall out with them. Christ, how I'd love to have a row with Mum and Dad or exchange a few cross words. But I can't. They are gone forever. If only people would just stop and think for a moment. You only get one Mum and Dad in life and who knows what the future holds. Yes there are circumstances that can never be resolved between a parent and a child. That's fair enough. However, I'm talking about the petty squabbles or the teenager that talks to their parents like a piece of shit. These can be resolved if people just make a little more effort.

Close you eyes and picture your own Mum or Dad.

Picture the good times. See them laughing, joking and smiling. Remember the last time they held you and told you that they loved you. I bet you are smiling and feel incredible warmth as you think of these happy memories. Now what if something happens to your Mum and Dad. There'll be no more happy times. No more laughing, joking and smiling. No more hugs and words of love. They are gone forever and the many years of happiness that you envisaged for the future are wiped out in an instant. Gone in a second.

I suppose what I am trying to say is spend more time with your Mum and Dad. Do things together before it's too late. Talk more and hug more. Otherwise you could end up feeling some serious guilt after they've gone and believe me it's not nice. I should know. Don't have any regrets.

There's no more I can say. That's enough. I can't write anymore on what it's like to lose a loved one to cancer. Christ, there's so much I haven't told you about my parents deaths, but to be honest these parts will remain private. They're too hard to talk about. If you've been through this awful scenario yourself, then you'll know what I'm talking about and I'm sure you'll understand. If you haven't, I truly hope that you don't have to watch someone you love go through such shit.

Right, that's it. I've finished and I can now put my pen down. Actually I'm knackered. I didn't realise that writing a book can leave you physically and mentally drained. However, it's been well worth it.

I can now look forward to becoming a Dad again very soon. I'll hold her in my arms and quietly whisper, "You're my little miracle from Daddy's one bollock."

What a cracking future I've got.

PS. if you are a lady who has just finished reading this book, then beware........................you are about to be shagged senseless by your other half! (Sorry, it's make love isn't it).